# BEYOND THE BUZZ

**Misty Lake**
**Beyond the Buzz**



Published by Spines Publishing Platform
ISBN: 979-8-90222-898-1

Spines

# BEYOND THE BUZZ

A MODERN GUIDE TO SMART CANNABIS USE

MISTY LAKE

## ENDORSEMENTS

A smart, stigma-busting walk through cannabis history, botany, ECS basics, and real-world use. Think "Cannabis 101" done cleanly—no woo, no lecturing, no pretension. A clean entry point for the canna-curious who want clarity without actually needing a PhD to follow along.

*~Jennifer Steinbachs, ND, PhD, Syringa Wellness, Sandpoint, ID*

"The information in this book is something I had been curious about for a long time, but I wasn't sure what information was trustworthy or useful. This book felt like the answer to that search. As someone who is aware of the limitations within the corporate medical and pharmaceutical system, I found it especially meaningful to learn about a more natural, holistic approach to healing—one that emphasizes understanding and balance rather than quick fixes."

*~ Paula Black, healing coach and author "Life, Cancer and God"*

"I loved the personal stories. I have similar stories about my own parents and introducing them to cbd. I also loved the story about how healing it has been for you and your dog. [I learned] so much, from the history to current political prohibition, and the dosage guide. I already want to share it with so many others. It was so informative and well written. It's going to become my new CBD bible."

~ *Jenny Simpkins, LMP, MMP, Body Revive, Cedar City, UT*

"Misty taught me so much about CBD. She presents a huge amount of information in a way that's easy to understand! I was hooked from page one thanks to the way she tells her story of overcoming the assumptions around CBD! She is truly a pioneer in the industry and a trailblazer for the healing effects of CBD!"

~ *Krysta Bell*

"It captured my attention from the very beginning. I look forward to referencing the book often."

~ *Cindy Ebel*

# DEDICATION

*This book was meant for you.*
*The nerds and the rebels.*
*The ones who strive to grow and heal.*
*The curious ones.*
*The experienced users.*
*The eager health advocates.*
*The lifelong learners. The crunchy ones.*
*The noobs and the original stoners.*
*The homesteaders and preppers.*
*The entrepreneurs.*
*The students. The creatives.*
*The cannabis industry—from the growers,*
*to delivery drivers to the budtenders.*
*The cannabis community—from corporations*
*to nonprofit organizations.*
*The medical community* ***AND***
*the anti-medical establishments.*

# CONTENTS

## NOTE TO READERS

The statements, stories, and topics discussed in this book are not FDA-approved, nor are they intended to diagnose, treat, cure, or prevent any diseases and/or disorders.

This book is for educational and entertainment purposes only. It is not intended to serve as medical advice. Please seek advice from your doctor or healthcare provider before adding any form of cannabis to your healthcare routine. Do not stop or change any prescription medications without your physician's guidance.

The author disclaims liability for any medical outcomes that may occur as a result of applying the methods discussed in this book.

# ACKNOWLEDGMENTS

This book has been a labor of love, and I want to thank God, first and foremost, for giving me the courage, skills, connections, and experiences to bring this book to life.

An extra special thank you to my husband, Scott, the love of my life. You are my favorite person, who is insanely intelligent. I couldn't have done this book without you. Not only did you nurture me through my health journey, but you also gave me the time, space, and support to explore and write about such a controversial topic—all of this while raising our two wonderful kiddos. I will always love and appreciate you.

I want to thank my kids for their endless encouragement. Keali and Eli, you both are so smart! You challenge and inspire me to be a better mom and person every day. Eli, you ask such thoughtful questions—many of which I answer in this book. Keali, I appreciate all of the talent and feedback you have provided during this writing process—from helping me create a cover image to designing many of the charts and illustrations for me. You truly are an integral part of the process! I wrote this book to encourage your generation and the generations to come to not only be open-minded but also *smart* about cannabis usage. Most importantly, be a leader, do your research, and make informed decisions. I love you both so much.

Another big thanks to Mom and Dad. My upbringing made me the person I am today. You raised Sis and me to be free thinkers, lifelong learners, independent, and self-reliant people. Thank you for allowing me to share some of the stories that helped shape this book. I would also like to thank my Sis, Crystal Pitts, who continues to inspire me. I am so proud of you!

Thank you, Shilo Vogel, Jenai Senteio, Gloria Lake, Chrissy Ragan, Shauna Shroeder, Ryan Smith, Misty Connella, Jennifer Steinbachs, Brandan Dunne, and Justin Dunne, for always believing in me. You all have been a constant source of inspiration and support in your own ways!

To Ryan and Donna McNamara, as well as Kylie and Tyler Nelsen, thank you for your continued hospitality during my cannabis education travels. Thanks to Crystal Smith for your contributions to the industry, research, and friendship. Thanks to Jenny Wiglesworth for giving me the opportunity to "test drive" my writing career. I will always appreciate you for taking a chance on my publishing career in your incredible magazine *People over Product.* Thank you for graciously being my editor. You gave me the confidence to follow through with the dream of publishing my own body of work.

A special thanks to Harold Robinson for taking me under your wing in the "corporate side" of the cannabis industry. A big thanks to all the retailers, collaborators, and customers of Herb 'N Oil. I learned so much about the business from you all. I appreciate all of the coaching clients, colleagues, and students with whom I have had the blessing to work over the years. I am also grateful for all the *Badass Bodyworkers* who sought answers and inspired me to learn more.

I am so grateful for the healthcare professionals, conference attendees, colleagues, friends, and family who encouraged me to share all of the "tidbits" of knowledge I have picked up along the journey. I want to thank those who have come before me and fought hard for the cannabis rights we are consistently gaining. Thank you to the herbalists, tribal elders, the healing arts community, and the growers for keeping the traditions and this ancient "sacred" plant medicine relevant.

Thanks to all who are a part of the research to further our knowledge about this incredible plant. Thank you to the activists, lobbyists, passionate parents, cannabis healthcare providers, educators, nonprofit groups, and alternative medical practices that continue to encourage safe, legal, and responsible usage.

Thank you, cannabis users, for creating a movement that can't be ignored. Last but not least, thank you to all the other writers in this genre and the authors in my life who have inspired me to share my own story and lessons.

# INTRODUCTION

In writing this book, I intend to share my personal journey with cannabis in order to help others along the same path of healing and bust some of the many myths that demonize this plant. Many in this field have experienced the dichotomy of cannabis. It can be a source of healing and controversy, hope and frustration, freedom and restriction. Perhaps the most surprising things I have learned about this fantastic plant lie in one of the most overlooked, undervalued components: the isolated cannabinoids, predominantly CBD (cannabidiol). The more you experience and learn about this beautiful plant, the more its potential is sure to astound you.

Sometimes, informational and self-help books can feel overwhelming. This is especially true when they get "science-y," like this one. For ease of use, I broke the book down into 4 parts in 20 chapters.

Part 1: Chapters 1–5

- Uncovering some of the sordid history of Cannabis in the USA, including tidbits on the "War on

Drugs" and the sad truth about the medical industry.
- Important updates to the legislation regarding hemp and busting popular myths about cannabis, marijuana, and hemp.

Part 2: Chapters 6–8

- Get to know the plant—from anatomy to the science behind CBD, THC, terpenes, and other cannabinoids.
- Learn about how and when cannabis testing is utilized and why it is important.
- Understand the types of processing that take the plant to market in its many forms.

Part 3: Chapters 9–16

- A crash course on the Endocannabinoid System (ECS)—how our bodies were designed to utilize this incredible plant.
- The biological differences between the ECS of men and women and what that means for usage.
- Cannabis (and non-cannabis) ways to support our ECS when it isn't functioning well
- Weighing the risks versus the rewards of THC usage and how to use it responsibly.

Part 4: Chapters 17–20

- Understanding dosing, labels, and common mistakes with using CBD
- Benefits that go with each type of CBD along with pros and cons.
- The truth about side effects, medication interactions, and what CBD can do for special populations.

Several of the chapters throughout the book include stories from my own life or from people I know. Sometimes, names will be changed in order to protect those who aren't comfortable revealing their identities.

### ***About Cannabis Research***

Important things to consider...

The date, the test subjects, the size, purpose, doses, and the parameters are all EXTREMELY important to consider and investigate when reading ANY research study.

Why are these things important?

- It may mean the difference between a product working or not working for you.
- It can also determine potential side effects, the length of time needed for the product to take effect, and even the optimal method of usage.

- The date and subjects can sometimes go hand in hand. (For example, in older studies, the law only allowed testing on rodents or petri dishes.)
- Various test subjects are still used in modern studies, but as we learn more about the human endocannabinoid system, we have discovered that there are important differences to note.

*For example: "...In contrast to rodent FAAH, CBD does not inhibit the enzymatic actions of human FAAH," according to a study published by the Journal of Biological Chemistry.*

Because of this difference, the study shows that CBD is an effective way to treat seizure disorders in humans but would be completely ineffective for treating them in mice.

- The purposes of these studies also vary greatly. It is easy to assume that the intention of many clinical studies is to find new medical or therapeutic uses, but another important mission is to assess the safety of a protocol or treatment.
- When the safety of a substance is studied, it can often be tested at extreme doses in order to understand the body's reaction to varying amounts.

# PART I

# OVERCOMING REEFER MADNESS & THE MARIJUANA STIGMA

## MYTHS BUSTED AND HISTORY UNCOVERED

# CHAPTER ONE

# HIGH IQ

Abraham Lincoln
Arnold Schwarzenegger
Barack Obama
Bill Gates
Carl Sagan
Christopher Columbus
Dave Chappelle
Elon Musk
George W. Bush
JFK
Joan of Arc
Ludwig van Beethoven
Maya Angelou
Marilyn Monroe
Michael Phelps
Morgan Freeman
Queen Victoria
Snoop Dogg
Steve Jobs
William Shakespeare

I am sure you recognize (at least some) of these names. Yes, they are all famous. They are influential. They are some of our world leaders. Some of them are innovators. All of them are leaving a legacy for the impact they have had on their own and future generations. Their names are scattered throughout the world in history books as artists, visionaries, athletes, revolutionaries, and inspirational figures. Each one has his or her own story that shaped the path that led them to greatness, just like you are shaping your story currently. They are (or were) highly intelligent people. Many of them are, or were, geniuses, and they all use (or used) cannabis.

Snoop Dogg smoking weed? This isn't a shocker, but did you know that he has an IQ of 147? Did you know that billionaire Elon Musk—undeniably a tech genius—has an IQ estimated to be between 155 and 160? He also publicly smoked a joint on "The Joe Rogan Experience," a popular podcast with over 19 million subscribers and billions of views. Every single person on this list has either professed to partake in, or there is evidence of their partaking in the controversial herb that has quickly gone from prohibition to exhibition in the last 13 years.

Although the above-mentioned individuals are on record for using some form of cannabis, that doesn't necessarily equate to "getting high." Not all cannabis products get you high. Both Hemp and medical cannabis containing high amounts of CBD are very popular within wealthy circles due to the powerful wellness benefits, along with the extremely negligible risks and side effects. "THC-Free Hemp CBD has especially become popular with those who have struggled with past substance abuse since it is non-addictive and non-intoxicating."

I have seen the use of cannabis enhance the thought processes, state of well-being, and mindset of many people throughout the years. Some of the smartest people I know (many of them true geniuses) use cannabis in some capacity or another, whether it's smoking a joint or using CBD on a daily basis.

Is cannabis use making them smarter?
Are smart people drawn to using cannabis?
If their use stopped, would they be even smarter?
Does it calm and focus the mind of someone with ADHD?
Does it open and expand the portal to creativity?

Can it create a "social buffer" for those who struggle to connect emotionally in relationships, crowds, or social gatherings?

Let me be the first to say that I am not a genius. I am just a lifelong learner and wellness nerd who loves to help others meet their full potential. There is so much more to learn about this plant and other healing herbs, how they interact with our bodies, the role that our past experiences play, and even how our current lifestyles influence our futures. I feel like cannabis is one of the many tools that hold the potential to aid many people along that journey. It may even help you.

On the flip side of that, I am not naive to the fact that there are still many states and countries where the use of even CBD is illegal, much less recreational forms of cannabis. I also know that in certain communities, black market cannabis is still rampant. Unless you are growing it yourself, it could easily be laced with dangerous substances and chemicals. For example, the risk of illegal weed being laced with fentanyl is very real, and I recently spoke to a young woman who was traumatized by experiencing this adulterated form. While low-THC hemp is a federally legal substance in the U.S., medical and recreational cannabis are still being regulated at a state level. As of early 2026, hemp has just recently become reclassified. It was federally regulated as a Class I drug (the same class as ecstasy and heroin), and President Trump just reclassified it, so now it is a Class III drug (now alongside ketamine and Tylenol with codeine).

I hope that by educating the general public about the potential benefits as well as risks, they will be better equipped to make responsible decisions as laws continue to change. I also hope readers can relate to and learn from some of my stories and experiences that changed my perspective on a lot more than just cannabis.

**I DARE you to think differently.**

Like many of you, I had a lot of trust in Western medicine as a kid and teen—so much, in fact, that I aspired to become a doctor one day. At the time, no one in my immediate family had graduated from college. Maybe I was different. I excelled academically; I loved to read and learn (and still do), and I was motivated to break the cycle of having a limited education that typically comes with a low-paying career.

My parents weren't hippies, despite the fact that they grew up during the stereotypical hippie movement of the '60s and '70s. I was born in the early '80s in Coeur d' Alene, Idaho. I grew up in a conservative, Christian, blue-collar household. My dad was an Air Force military police officer turned career concrete contractor. My mom, despite her struggle with fibromyalgia, which you'll read more about later, also worked full-time while raising my sister and me. We all pitched in to care for our 5-acre ranch, which consisted mostly of rabbits and exotic pheasants. The ranch also included chickens, turkeys, ducks, horses, goats, and dogs.

I was a 4-H kid who rode horses with Mom, went fishing with Dad, showed chickens and bunnies at the local fair, and was raised on homegrown beef. Along with beef, our diets consisted of free-range chickens, fresh-caught lake trout, venison, and an abundance of berries and vegetables from our massive garden. It was a humble and wholesome upbringing that I truly took for granted in my childhood.

My father was, and still is, a stickler for the rules and was a devoted news watcher. He "ate it all up" like many of his peers. The moment the "war on drugs" was in full swing, he quickly jumped on board and saw it as a teaching opportunity for my sister and me as we entered our teen years.

He'd tell us stories about getting harassed on the basketball courts by the "druggies and stoners" who hung out in Yuma, Arizona, during his formative years. They would frequently bully him, the tall and lanky high schooler with the thick-rimmed glasses. Later in life, as an entrepreneur, he struggled to find motivated employees who didn't smoke weed on their lunch breaks, only to have to pick up their slack at work. These actions only solidified his stance on the harms of substance abuse. I felt for him, but I also questioned what specific drugs these guys were on, as my experience with stoners was vastly different.

I grew up in the 90s era of Drug Abuse Resistance Education (*DARE*). I had been a card-carrying, DARE t-shirt-wearing member since the 6th grade. Like many others in my middle and high school, I bought into the idea of the "This is your brain on drugs" frying pan ad that frequented our screens during prime-time TV commercial breaks. I was indoctrinated to believe that if you used drugs, you likely wouldn't finish high school—much less go to college. You would presumably end up working at McDonald's for the rest of your life (no offense to those who work there—it just wasn't something I was aspiring to do).

D.A.R.E. tried to make this indoctrination "fun." There were coloring books, logoed gear (including fancy pens, bumper stickers, etc.). Their intentions were seemingly good. They provided drug education, talked about leading a healthy lifestyle, encouraged communication with trusted adults, and empowered us to "just say no!" to peer pressure through role-playing and case studies.

I also enjoyed the fact that we "DARE kids" got to participate in drug-free activities at a drastically reduced price—sometimes even for free. Coming from limited means, this was a HUGE perk for my friends and me, who resided in the lower income brackets. These activities and events included group gatherings such as skiing, snowboarding, pizza parties, movies, and skate nights at the local roller rink. These outings were often accompanied by 1-2 local "DARE officers" who encouraged and reminded us to resist peer pressure and to basically become informants for the department by practicing the 3 R's: Recognize, Resist, and Report if we saw someone using drugs or found drugs in our homes.

The program's goals were tied to resisting other unsavory influences as well, such as joining a gang, engaging in violence, and partaking in the destruction of property (graffiti, bashing mailboxes, breaking windows, etc.). We were told that all these things were intrinsically linked and that "doing drugs was the root cause to all of it."

As my friend group expanded through the middle school and high school years, I started to realize that many of my friends were doing some of these "awful things." They were smoking cigarettes, drinking alcohol, and even smoking weed. However, they were still achieving good grades and not joining gangs. They still had ambitious futures that they were working toward while holding part-time jobs, volunteering, and earning scholarships.

Could the law enforcement and media have been lying to us? Was drinking a beer REALLY as dangerous as snorting a line of cocaine? Was smoking a joint REALLY the gateway to a heroin overdose? I truly felt deceived, confused, and frustrated. What else have they been lying about? Was I missing something? I had yet to see the connection—the downward spiral that we were led to believe was inevitable.

Here I am, entering my "rebellious" teen years, and I discover through personal observation that the "role models," aka DARE officers, had not been telling us the full truth. Although I knew that there was some *semblance of truth* to the dangers of drug and alcohol use, it didn't fully add up based on my experiences. I had seen way more harm done by alcohol use vs. marijuana, yet it was socially and culturally acceptable—and even encouraged in social settings.

I had seen a grandpa succumb to liver cancer in his mid-50s after a lifetime of heavy cigarette smoking and alcoholism. I had lost peers to drunk drivers and alcohol-induced liver failure. I knew the impact of alcoholism on a family. I had heard of all the stories of celebrity drug overdoses and news reports on drugs. Most of them centered around increased gang violence on the West Coast among teens.

I had no desire to shoot up, join a gang, or make drinking a daily habit. I did, however, start questioning the impact of alcohol use, though. Was even occasional use safe? What about marijuana? I didn't know ANYONE that smoked pot at the time who would say, "That was awesome! Now, I really want crack!" On top of which, I don't recall anyone having ANY negative health effects or having done harm to others due to cannabis usage.

It actually just made me curious. Healthcare had always interested me, and I wanted to learn more. So, like many teens in the '90s who grew up in the Pacific Northwest listening to Green Day, Nirvana, and Stone Temple Pilots, I experimented with smoking pot at an occasional bonfire on the mountain or at a house party on the prairie.

I didn't love it. Nor did I hate it. Cannabis really didn't become part of my life until later on down the road. That particular path didn't seem to fit in with the fact that I wanted to become a doctor—or so I thought at the time.

Maybe your background was similar, but even if it wasn't, I encourage you to keep an open mind about cannabis. You may be surprised at the history of cannabis prohibition—how it threatens our current medical system and how it could truly be the missing piece of preventative medicine that could reverse the damage our current system has caused.

Never in my wildest dreams would I imagine myself writing a book on cannabis, becoming a public speaker, or educating people about it. I had no clue that it would eventually save the lives of many people whom I know and care about. I wouldn't have ever fathomed that it would give me MY LIFE back.

## CHAPTER TWO

# MY BAD, I THOUGHT DOCTORS... HEALED PEOPLE.

By the time we are adults, most people in the U.S. have had some experience with doctors, hospitals, or other Western medical practices. They get us started early on with childhood vaccinations, annual exams, sports physicals, and flu shots—all prior to being "sick or injured" and all in the name of "preventive medicine."

I know that not everyone is afforded the "luxury" of these services. There are many underserved populations. Many families ride the fine line between not qualifying for Medicaid and not being able to afford health insurance. Nor do they have easy access to the providers that serve these populations (even with the "Affordable Care Act"). Not everyone believes these services are necessary, or even actually preventative—but we won't go there; that is a story for another book.

Experience with the U.S. medical system can vary greatly from person to person. Maybe you had ear infections or a broken bone as a child. Perhaps you needed stitches or a tetanus shot. Or maybe your healthcare experience was not about you at all. It is possible you had a parent or sibling with health issues, and the hospital was your second home. Maybe your experience was on the other side of the equation, and you grew up with medical professionals in the family. No matter your experience, you likely have an opinion about the healthcare system of the U.S. This has especially been a hot topic since 2020 due to the conflicting information that arose from the COVID-19 pandemic.

We are incredibly blessed here in the USA to have some AMAZING life-saving medical interventions, as well as highly educated professionals practicing modern medicine. I truly believe that every person and situation is unique when it comes to healthcare needs.

I also believe that nothing is black and white. Yes, Western medicine can be a blessing. I am not bashing doctors here, just frustrated with the system. Yes, modalities such as Traditional Chinese Medicine, Ayurveda, and alternative therapies, such as herbal medicine and energy work, are also amazing. They were the "original" forms of healthcare, and I feel like too much of those traditions, as well as indigenous medicine, have been unnecessarily abandoned in the Western world.

I believe a highly effective healthcare system would incorporate the best of BOTH worlds. In order for change to happen, however, there needs to be a higher awareness of the problems. This includes the *truth* about the untapped potential in plant medicine that has been hidden from the public eye due to greed and fear tactics.

* * *

***Fun Fact:***

Did you know that in 1937, Cannabis was removed from the U.S. Pharmacopeia? The U.S. Pharmacopeia (USP) was a non-profit founded in 1820 that set the standard formulations for both human and animal medicine and supplements that were considered safe and effective. Cannabis was added to this book in 1850, but evidence of worldwide historical usage dates back to 5,000 years prior in what is known as the country of Romania. (More on this in "U.S. Cannabis History & Deceit" in ch. 6.)

* * *

I started seeing the red flags, even as a child. Growing up with a parent (my mom) who has chronic pain allowed me to see a side of the medical industry that I think most children aren't necessarily aware of. My curiosity led me to accompany her to several appointments throughout the years—MRIs, CAT scans, ultrasounds—and to see specialists. It was fascinating, scary, frustrating, and amazing—all at once.

I was curious about the technology and the inner workings of the human body. I was impressed by the sheer knowledge of the different types of procedures and testing. I also felt frustrated for my mom, who was STILL getting little to no answers as to why she was in constant pain.

Practically every new trip to the doctor's office or hospital produced another new medication. Sometimes they worked, but usually not well enough to compensate for the extreme side effects she dealt with from taking them. When one wouldn't work, they would prescribe her a new one, followed by running more tests. This cycle repeated over and over again. NSAIDs, SSRIs, corticosteroids, opioids, and benzos—more often than not, these prescriptions would be combined, sometimes in lieu of the previous ones that didn't work. This cycle continued for YEARS. She tried physical therapy, which caused even more bodily pain. She had surgeries that helped some of the issues, but often the relief was only temporary.

She eventually got diagnosed with fibromyalgia and began seeing a new doctor, who suggested massage therapy. She was cautiously optimistic since, at least, it was non-invasive. Even if it didn't help much, at least it wouldn't do any long-term damage like some of the meds she had tried.

Massage therapy actually brought her relief! After her first therapeutic massage session, she was sore for a couple of days. However, for several days following that, she felt SO MUCH BETTER. As her appointments became more regular, so did her relief—for longer periods of time.

I thought, "Weird, why hadn't any of the other doctors suggested this?" Well, massage therapy addresses key drivers of healthcare spending—chronic pain, stress-related conditions, musculoskeletal disorders, and reliance on medication—by improving function, reducing perceived pain, and supporting nervous system regulation.

During that same time period, when I was in my teens, I had numerous personal experiences with the inadequacies of our healthcare system. During high school, I dislocated my knee (ouch!). After X-rays, an orthopedic surgeon consultation, and a LOT of physical therapy, I was told that not only should I never run again, but surgery was inevitable. There were several chunks of cartilage that broke off during my injury, and the pieces were now floating around underneath my kneecap. These chunks would occasionally get lodged between my femur and tibia, and I couldn't bend my leg. There was zero discussion or thought about why a healthy and active 17-year-old would be at risk for a full subluxation of a strong joint by casually dancing in the first place. **Side note: I lifted weights under the supervision of an experienced trainer 3-5 days a week, did cardio regularly, and danced almost daily as a varsity cheerleader. I wasn't exactly out of shape. Sadly, I was given no advice or suggestions on how to prevent it from happening again beyond "Go to PT and don't run." This was extremely frustrating.

Within a year, I wound up injuring my shoulder in a car accident. Even though I was sent to the hospital and "checked out," which included a physical exam and X-rays, they simply gave me pain meds and sent me straight to physical therapy. It was VERY painful to even attempt a majority of the movements that they required. I couldn't physically do anything that required me to lift my elbow more than 90 degrees away from my body. Even on painkillers, I choked back tears during every treatment, telling them that it wasn't working. They just kept repeating, "It's just the swelling. The strain just needs to heal."

Roughly two weeks into PT, I was helping my mom with some laundry when I heard and felt a *POP!!* My shoulder found its home—back in the socket where it belonged. My full range of motion returned instantly, and I was relieved. Although I was a bit sore, I was mostly mad at the torture that I had been put through. I was also confused as to why this wasn't caught sometime during the ER visit, at the doctor's office when they read the X-ray, or at any of the other six PT appointments.

On multiple other occasions during high school, I fainted. The ER staff would tell me I was "dehydrated" again, pump me with IV fluids, and send me on my way. They never believed me when I told them I was drinking enough water. They didn't run tests or question why a physically fit high school girl who ate whole, clean foods, plenty of vegetables and protein, and got good sleep was landing in the ER so frequently.

By the time I graduated high school in '99, I had also earned my CNA (Certified Nursing Assistant) and MA (Medical Assistant) certificates, allowing me to work in healthcare right away. This was before starting the pre-med program in which I was enrolled at Oregon State

University. It really didn't take long before I began to understand the role that capitalism played in our medical industry.

It is easy to forget that hospitals and medical practices are businesses until you work in one. I saw and experienced the way that the health insurance industry dictated medical treatments for many patients who are not informed about their "other options." I also became keenly aware of the fact that most people don't want to do any form of "work" to improve their health—they just expect to be "fixed." Because of this, patient adherence and compliance can be extremely low for treatment plans that involve taking responsibility for their own well-being. This would include activities such as exercising daily or even simply drinking adequate amounts of water.

It made me realize three major flaws in our healthcare system:

1. A large majority of physicians are hesitant to become patient advocates due to potential employer retaliation and backlash from not maintaining "neutrality." It can also become time-prohibitive and challenging in certain settings.
2. Doctors are not paid to "heal" you—only to diagnose and treat. MANY times, with the exception of trauma care, these things do not actually lead to "healing," only to symptom management.

3. Preventative health measures (nutrition, exercise, mental health, and sleep) are up to the doctor's discretion, and they are taught very little in med school: roughly 1% of the curriculum is about diet and nutrition. More than half of graduated physicians have not received ANY formal training about exercise, as it is only an elective. An average of under 2.5 hours of doctors' education is spent on sleep, with roughly 27% responding that they didn't receive ANY sleep education (according to a study done by the NIH).

During my undergrad pre-med program and real-world experience, I had learned enough about Western medicine, addiction, Big Pharma, and the role (or lack thereof) of holistic healthcare in Western society that I decided I didn't want to continue down that path. As a young adult, through travel and meeting people from different cultures, my mind had become more open to the unique traditions and practices of self-care and natural health that aren't in "mainstream" medicine in the U.S. I fell in love with massage therapy in 2002 and graduated from massage school in 2003.

I naturally gravitated to clinical work and took ongoing training certifications to focus on chronic pain, oncology massage, advanced medical massage, and palliative care clients. My medical massage career was rewarding. I felt incredibly blessed to be collaborating with so many alternative medicine providers who truly advocated for their patients and achieved real results by addressing the underlying root causes of health issues.

In 2009, I ended up moving only 90 minutes away from my hometown in North Idaho to Washington State. It was the first state, along with Colorado, to pass the law for legal recreational cannabis in 2012.

The nation was eagerly watching to see how these new laws would affect everything from cannabis use in minors to driving while intoxicated, workplace accidents, and opioid abuse.

- Would the additional tax income be significant?
- How many people would it draw who are seeking more freedom for medical use?
- Would it boost the economy, or create a lazy and unmotivated workforce?
- Would it cut down on "unclean" or "black market" weed?

The cannabis demand in Eastern Washington had grown exponentially. My medical massage clients were predominantly palliative care patients seeking alternative therapies. Many had already been using medical marijuana or were ready to learn more due to the new legal status. (*Side note: Medical marijuana was passed in 1998 in Washington.)*

The clients who were already medical cannabis users had shared their journeys. Some had no hesitation diving into herbal medicine because it was natural. Others, however, felt like it was a "last-ditch effort" to potentially extend their time left. I heard stories of miracles—MANY miracles. The common thread among these survivors was never just cannabis.

It was a mindset.
Faith.
Hope.
Support.
It was usually a complete change in lifestyle.
Often giving up high stress
jobs/relationships/living situations/environments
in lieu of embracing the things that TRULY MATTER.
Letting go of guilt, shame, and resentments, and
forgiving themselves and others
who have caused trauma and emotional turmoil.
It was paying attention to their bodies.
Becoming conscious of what they ate, drank, thought, and
how they spent their time and energy.
It was prioritizing the people in their lives that mattered
and loving to the fullest.

They were and are inspiring. They reminded me that you don't have to get sick or be on your deathbed to create positive changes in your life. Cannabis was just a tool in their arsenal—like good sleep and clean water. I needed to find out what made this plant so special and unique.

Starting in 2013, I tapped into various local resources, reaching out to growers I knew for more information on the subject. I began researching the therapeutic benefits of cannabis in order to help people navigate the new laws. I hoped to help people understand that certain types of cannabis were more beneficial for certain conditions than others when used for palliative care.

Many of my clients knew that I made all my own massage oils and were willing to be my "guinea pigs" when I started infusing my oils with CBD-dominant cannabis. They were using it for joint pain, muscle recovery, surgical healing, skin conditions, cancer, and more.

As my massage clients continued to get incredible results, I kept modifying the recipe to improve the efficacy, smell, and absorption. All the while, I was in constant research mode—reading worldwide clinical studies in relation to conditions, usage, individual cannabinoids, terpenes, and how the body processes it all in the endocannabinoid system. It was FASCINATING! I was so excited to share my new passion with my family.

I got so excited to tell my mom about the results that my fibromyalgia clients were experiencing—hoping that she, too, could try it out. When we started the conversation, though, she quickly stated, "I wouldn't say anything to Dad about this." She was on board for trying it for her own conditions but wanted to keep it on the down low.

Ugh! Didn't Dad know that times have changed? I mean, with as much news as he watched, hasn't he seen the legislation changing all over the country? Doesn't he realize that medical marijuana is now legal in most states? I really just wanted to explain the benefits of CBD to him and make him realize how therapeutic and safe its usage is.

Ignoring my mom's advice, I brought the subject up the next time I saw him. This was a bad idea. His temper flared, and he refused to listen to anything I had to say on the subject. Case closed.

# CHAPTER THREE

# "CANNABIS" VS. "MARIJUANA" VS. "HEMP"

## The 2014 Farm Bill

The U.S. finally modifies the Agricultural Law to allow hemp production for limited research purposes under state-operated pilot programs with limited federal oversight.

I was now on a mission to help people understand how our bodies are designed to utilize cannabis, how it threatens Western medicine, the history of why the government is controlling this iconic plant, and to bust the common myths about it.

This was a HUGE step in the right direction for the USA, but unfortunately, they were still leagues behind other developed nations when it came to research, acceptance, and usage of hemp for both industrial and medicinal purposes. When I got all excited about this, people started asking me why. Some of their questions were:

What was the difference between marijuana and hemp?
If hemp can't get you high,
Why does it matter whether it is legal or not?
Is hemp the same as cannabis?

Is it the same as marijuana?
What is the difference between the three?

Regardless of the federal legality of hemp, it was still considered a "gray area" in the eyes of the law when it came to individual state legislatures. This was, and still can be, confusing for many people.

## Cannabis vs. Marijuana vs. Hemp

It is easy to confuse the various terms for this amazing plant, so let's just start with the basics. All three terms are cannabis. "Cannabis," "marijuana," and "hemp" are terms often used to describe different classifications based on attributes of the same plant. The main differences between them lie in their uses, chemical composition, and legal statuses.

## Cannabis

Definition: Cannabis is a genus of flowering plants that includes various species, the most common being Cannabis sativa, Cannabis indica, and Cannabis ruderalis. It is the overarching term that describes ALL of the different types of plants, including medical marijuana, hemp, and recreational cannabis (aka marijuana, weed, pot, dope, ganja, reefer, etc.).

Legalities may vary based on THC content and location.

- Cannabis that is classified as "hemp" is federally legal in the USA but is state-regulated and varies

from state to state, regardless of the federal stance.
- Cannabis that is classified as "medical use" (aka medical marijuana or medical cannabis) is also state-regulated and is still illegal in a few U.S. states, varying by state.
- Recreational Use Cannabis is federally illegal in the U.S., but it is legal and regulated in other countries such as Canada. European laws are not only location-dependent but can also be product-dependent. Within the U.S., recreational cannabis is regulated at the state level as well, with some states opting to legalize use for adults over the age of 21 with state-specific laws and rules.

Uses: Cannabis plants can be cultivated for various purposes, including industrial uses, medicinal applications, and recreational use (to relieve pain and provide other benefits while becoming intoxicated).

Chemical Composition: Cannabis plants contain a range of compounds called cannabinoids, with delta-9-tetrahydrocannabinol (THC) and cannabidiol (CBD) being the most well-known. The cannabinoids CBG, CBN, delta-8, and CBC, as well as other constituents of the plant, are quickly emerging as promising therapeutic components in the marketplace.

Prior to cannabis prohibition in the 1930s, Cannabis was the scientific term used in apothecaries and pharmacies.

"Hemp" was either called hemp for general industrial uses or "psychoactive hemp," a term used for anyone who utilized any form of hemp outside industrial uses, regardless of the THC percentage.

**Marijuana**

*Can be either "Recreational Cannabis" or "Medical Cannabis."*

Definition: "Marijuana" is a term used to describe the Cannabis sativa or Cannabis indica plant when it is cultivated for its psychoactive properties, meaning it has active THC. The term "marijuana" is a bit archaic and can be considered derogatory due to the history associated with it. More on that in "US Cannabis History & Deceit" at the end of Chapter 6. For clarity, throughout the book, I will use the terms "Recreational Cannabis" or "Medicinal Cannabis" to specify their intended purposes.

Uses and Chemical Composition: Marijuana is primarily used for its recreational and medicinal effects.

It is consumed for the euphoric "high" induced by THC. Marijuana plants are bred to have higher THC levels, which can range from moderate to high, depending on the strain or type.

> ***Medical marijuana*** is a Cannabis plant that provides benefits for patients looking for enhanced pain relief balanced with the therapeutic effects of CBD.
> Legalities: It is regulated by the government and

may require a prescription, registration, and/or license to obtain or grow. Its chemical composition typically includes BOTH CBD and THC in significant amounts in order to have enhanced medicinal value.

***Recreational marijuana*** is a Cannabis plant that is bred to have a higher (pun intended) THC content in order to provide users with a strong euphoric effect that can range from uplifted, energetic creativity to "couch lock," a deeply relaxed and/or "chill" state.
Legalities: As of early 2026, cannabis has been legalized for recreational purposes for those aged 21 and older in 24 states and 3 U.S. territories. Some states carry products for purchase in dispensaries or retail stores. Others, however, allow you to grow your own. Still, others allow a combination of the two. Typically, there is little to no CBD in recreational cannabis. However, depending on your location's laws, there may be some crossover in what types of marijuana are carried at dispensaries.

## Hemp

Definition: Hemp refers to a variety of the Cannabis sativa plant that is cultivated for either industrial and/or therapeutic purposes. In most legal documentation (at least in the U.S.), all hemp is categorized as industrial.

Legalities: The definition of hemp varies by country since it is actually a legal classification based on the percentage of THC per dry weight.

In the US, the federal definition for hemp puts it at .3% (more on the details in More Legal Stuff, the 2018 Farm Bill. Since Hemp does not have enough THC in it to intoxicate you in its natural state, it is increasingly becoming legalized or decriminalized in many western and eastern countries.

Hemp-derived CBD products can be found in a wide variety of retail locations as well as online. There are still states that closely regulate the federally legal hemp CBD products, so it is important to check your local laws.

Uses:

> ***Industrial Hemp*** is grown for a multitude of uses outside of its therapeutic applications. When cultivated for its fibers or bast, it is grown closely spaced outdoors and left unpruned to prevent branching. It is often also grown for height and harvested prior to the flowering stage.
> If grown for seeds and hemp seed oil, they are still grown similarly; in this case, they will be producing flowers. The males and females grow together in order to promote open pollination and fertilization of the females to produce seeds.
> They are specifically bred for their intended purpose

—be it seed or bast (for fibers, fuel, etc.). Industrial hemp is used in the production of textiles, paper, biofuels, food products, and various industrial applications.

***Therapeutic Hemp*** (the flower of the female hemp plant) is used for herbal medicine. This dates back centuries and has re-emerged in Western culture as its dominant cannabinoid, CBD, is now a mainstream supplement.
Hemp is bred and cultivated for its cannabinoid content much like medical and recreational cannabis. In fact, if you saw them side by side, you wouldn't be able to differentiate them. Since CBD medical research has come a long way and is, in my opinion, highly undervalued, this is the main focus of this book.
Chemical Composition: Hemp has low THC levels (below 0.3%) - the psychoactive compound responsible for the "high" associated with marijuana. Its predominant active cannabinoid is CBD (cannabidiol) which is non-intoxicating.

The legal status of these terms varies worldwide, with hemp often being legal due to its industrial uses and low THC content, while all marijuana is subject to legal restrictions. However, all forms of cannabis are still illegal in the Middle East, Russia, several South American countries, and in a majority of African countries. Be sure to check the local and international laws before traveling with ANY cannabis products, including hemp.

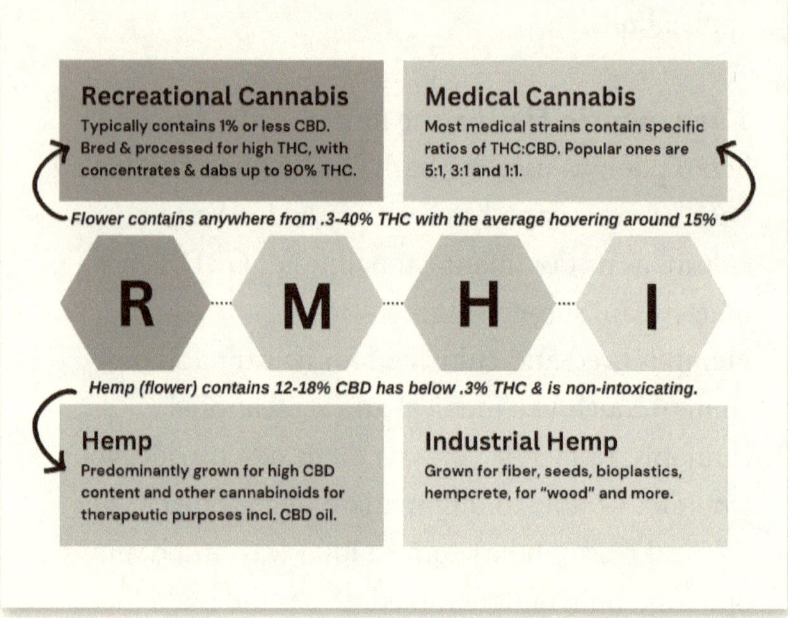


"In summary, while 'cannabis' is the overarching term for the plant, 'hemp' is a specific variety cultivated for industrial purposes with low THC content. 'Medical cannabis' is cultivated for the combined therapeutic effects of both THC and CBD. 'Recreational cannabis' includes plants cultivated for their psychoactive effects with higher THC levels."

# CHAPTER FOUR

# LAWS, DECEIT, AND MISCONCEPTIONS

## 2015 - Idaho - the "THC Free" state... not to be confused with Iowa.

The opportunity presented itself to allow my husband, kids, and me to move back to our hometown of Coeur d' Alene, Idaho in the summer of 2015. This move opened the doors to a whole new realm of opportunities and challenges.

Only a couple of months after moving homes, practices, and schools, I was rear-ended in my car on the freeway. Restarting my medical massage business in the new location had to be put on hold while I took the time to heal.

Fortunately, my soft-tissue injuries didn't hold me down for too long, but they did clue me in that there was something "not right" about my health, even though the doctors had cleared me to return to work. Even with the utilization of chiropractic care, physical therapy, and massage therapy, I was thankful to have CBD massage oils during my recovery process. The oils helped ease the aches and pains of healing from the car accident.

At this point, only 4 states had recreational cannabis legalized: Washington, Colorado, Oregon, and Alaska. Twenty-three states, plus the District of Columbia, had some form of medical marijuana laws in place. Many states, at this time, had been in the process of making modifications to their laws in order to allow hemp CBD usage. A few states placed specific limitations, restrictions, and regulations on Hemp CBD.

Now that I was in Idaho, ALL THC was illegal unless it was prescribed for children with uncontrolled epilepsy. Even if it was derived from the hemp plant- which meant that it had less than .3% THC dry weight, which is not enough to get you high. The Idaho office of drug policy went even further to specify that the "CBD must both contain zero THC and be derived from one of the five identified parts of the cannabis plant, otherwise it is illegal in Idaho".

This would mean I would have to use a pre-processed form of hemp, purchased outside the state of Idaho. The oil would have to come from specific parts of the plant, but not the flower, even though that was where CBD was most abundant. It would also have to go through a specific extraction process in order to remove any THC.

They did this by first making it into a concentrated form of oil, then removing (referred to as remediation or remediating) the THC, leaving behind a broad-spectrum extract. Although the broad-spectrum product sounded legal based on the fact that it was THC-free, Idaho law further specified that it also must not contain the "resin extracted from any part of such plant."

To accomplish this, one would extract the CBD entirely from the biomass, the non-flower plant parts, to avoid utilizing restricted plant parts or resin. This produced a dry, off-white powder that is 99+% pure isolated CBD, often referred to as "CBD Isolate" or "Pharmaceutical-grade CBD" (which we will discuss in more depth later).

At this time, there was a pharmaceutical solution called Epidiolex® that was made from CBD isolate and used for treating seizures associated with Lennox-Gastaut syndrome, Dravet syndrome, or Tuberous Sclerosis Complex (TSC) in patients aged one and older.

The restrictions set forth by Idaho laws ended up being an unexpected blessing. Due to my obsessive research, I learned SO MUCH MORE about CBD than I ever anticipated. CBD in its isolated form, quickly became the primary cannabinoid I turned to for the health of myself and my family.

In 2016, I opened a new massage clinic that had a modest Hemp CBD retail section in Post Falls, Idaho. I offered THC-free CBD massage regularly, and with clients' consent, I educated them along the way. My business grew quickly, and I realized that I needed to build a team in order to serve my community. As I hired massage therapists and other staff members to run the clinic, I taught them about the benefits, laws, and limitations surrounding the hemp CBD industry.

Because of the laws in Idaho being so strict about hemp, I was constantly being questioned about the legality of the products I was using. It gave me the opportunity to educate others about the intricacies of Idaho hemp law, as well as the differences between what I was using, making, and selling versus the CBD oil that was sold and legal in Washington State just over the border (from medical cannabis) or online (e.g., full-spectrum hemp CBD oil). Although selling CBD oil was legal federally, it was still extremely restrictive in a few states, including Idaho.

People typically thought that CBD oil either got you high or didn't work at all. I continually felt like I was swimming upstream. Explaining the endocannabinoid system, teaching the differences between internal use and external use, coaching practitioners and healthcare professionals on usage and interactions for their patients, and discussing these things with law enforcement felt like a full-time job. I wanted to help them understand what the lab results looked like for legal products vs. illegal (in Idaho). This became a consuming part of my practice.

Over the next couple of years, I continued to learn, create new products, and educate those around me. The training and consulting extended to my peers in the massage industry to local and national retailers who wanted to sell my products. After this, it then spread to groups of healthcare professionals across the U.S., who were receiving mixed information from the media and the pharmacists, who weren't very keen on a product with so little regulation and (U.S., double-blind, human) clinical studies.

There was a lot of research out there in other countries, and the U.S. was VERY slow to catch up. Luckily, the 2018 Farm Bill aimed to change this.

## More Legal Stuff: The 2018 Farm Bill

In 2018, a NEW Farm Bill was enacted to replace the 2014 one called the Agriculture Improvement Act of 2018. It addressed several aspects of US Nutrition and Agriculture programs that were in dire need of updating. The new, redefined legislation was incredibly important for the hemp industry in five major ways.

1. Legalization of Industrial Hemp: The bill removed hemp from the list of controlled substances, legalizing the cultivation, production, and distribution of industrial hemp. This marked a significant shift for the industry, allowing farmers to grow hemp for various purposes, including textiles, paper, food (hemp seeds and hemp seed oil), and CBD (cannabidiol) extraction.

2. Definition of Hemp: The legislation defined hemp as cannabis plants with a THC (tetrahydrocannabinol) content of 0.3% or less on a dry weight basis. This distinction differentiates hemp from marijuana, which has higher THC levels and remains a controlled substance.

3. Access to Federal Crop Insurance: Hemp producers gained access to federal crop insurance, providing them with a safety net against potential losses from natural disasters or other common unforeseen circumstances. This was a crucial step in supporting hemp cultivation as a legitimate agricultural crop.

4. Research Opportunities: The Farm Bill expanded opportunities for hemp research, allowing institutions of higher education and state departments of agriculture to conduct research and pilot programs related to hemp cultivation.

5. Interstate Commerce: This legislation enabled the legal transport of hemp and hemp products across state lines. It also facilitated the growth of the industry by opening up broader markets for hemp-derived goods.

Overall, these provisions aimed to stimulate the growth of the hemp industry, promote research, and provide a regulatory framework for its development within the broader agricultural landscape. These guidelines opened up commerce for a myriad of industries. Unfortunately, there was no regulatory agency specifically established (or even industry standards at this point) to act as a safety or protective measure for producers and consumers. It became an open market for anyone who wanted to cash in on the "legal" hemp craze. Companies started cashing in on the ignorance of the general public regarding all things hemp, causing all sorts of misinformation to arise about the industry.

***Hemp Myth #1: "I have CBD in my hemp seed oil."***

***Reality: There is NO CBD in hemp seed oil.***

CBD can be derived from ANY cannabis plant (hemp or medical marijuana, and even some recreational strains) that has CBD in its genetics. CBD is most abundantly found in the flower/bud of the female plant. Small amounts of CBD are also found in the leaves, and an even smaller amount is found in the stems and stalks. There is NO CBD in the seeds or roots of the plant, despite popular belief. This means that there is no CBD in hemp seed oil. I must make this clear for SO MANY reasons.

There are retailers out there selling "CBD oil" that is ONLY made with hemp seed oil. Because of this, customers are getting discouraged and, frankly, ripped off. In 2025, the average price per ounce for each was as follows:

Hemp seed oil: $0.60–$1.30/oz

CBD oil: $30–$200+/oz

You do the math. It is easy to see how someone can buy a gallon (128 oz) of hemp seed oil for $85 and rebottle it into 1 oz dropper bottles. They market it as "CBD Oil," resell the 1 oz bottles for $15-$25 wholesale, and retailers turn around and sell at $30-$100+ each retail. That is a MASSIVE profit on straight-up deception. Customers are expecting the healing benefits of CBD oil but are only getting the nutritional benefits from the omega fatty acids of hemp seed oil.

Common uses for CBD oil include powerful anti-inflammatory benefits, mental health support, nervous system regulation, immune system response regulation, gut health improvement, reproductive health enhancement, pain relief, treatment of skin conditions, alleviation of muscle aches, cell regeneration, boosting collagen production, and more (discussed in Chapter 7).

Common uses for hemp seed oil include cooking—providing a boost of omega-6 and omega-3 fatty acids—and skincare, as an antioxidant-rich moisturizer. Those who have been misled to believe that hemp seed oil contains CBD are now either claiming that CBD is "snake oil," believing it is a scam, or they believe that CBD oil "works," but just not for them. Both of which couldn't be further from the truth.

It is so unfortunate that these things happen. There are some companies out there that have good intentions and truly want to help those in need, but they have been misled by someone who was misinformed. However, other companies are doing this on purpose, cashing in on the trends—intentionally mislabeling and marketing these products in order to make a quick buck (and sometimes to skirt regulations).

On a federal level, the cannabis industry is considered a high-risk business. It can be difficult for most companies to not only get banking and credit card processing, but there is also a LOT of red tape to go through and restrictions on marketing cannabis products, including CBD since it is not (as of this writing) regulated by the FDA. This presents challenges that hemp seed oil doesn't have since it doesn't actually contain CBD. I have seen it both ways.

So don't forget, whenever looking at CBD products (especially on Amazon and in many big box stores), keep in mind that *there is NO CBD in hemp seed oil.*

## "Bananas and Deceit"

It was February of 2018 on Maui, and the "bananas were ripe for the picking." As the women of my family prepped for the wedding, the men were doing their best to be productive while staying out of the way.

The father of the bride, a.k.a. my dad, noticed the nearby trees strained under the weight of the familiar yellow fruit, introduced to the islands in the 1800s. My dad caught the attention of my soon-to-be brother-in-law.

"Happy to harvest some bananas for you so they don't drop and attract the rodents. I just need something to cut them down with," my dad mentioned hopefully.

In just a mere few minutes, my dad was eagerly sawing away at the base of a banana bunch that was hanging up near the top of the tree—at what was easily over twice his height. Not being a wasteful person, he was concerned about the ripe fruit bruising as it dropped from such a significant height. As the bunch began to creak and droop under its own weight, he quickly dropped the tree-pruning tool and reached out to catch the bundle of ripe fruit in his arms before it dropped to the soft, tropical turf.

"AAaaghh!!" My father's booming baritone shout rang across the bay.

He heard the snap and felt the agony of the 50+ lbs. banana bunch rip his biceps right off the bone. I can't imagine the excruciating pain he felt. Two surgeries, three weeks, and lots of appointments with the VA later, he was really struggling with pain management. He had been back home in cold and snowy Idaho and was already starting to rehab his arm and shoulder. Along with the torn bicep tendons, the catch had dislocated his shoulder and broken his wrist. He probably should have just let those bananas bruise a little, I thought. As a former massage therapist and his daughter, I hated seeing him in pain.

As I was saying in Chapter 2, my dad was NOT happy about the CBD side gig I had started alongside my medical massage clinic several years back. It ended up organically morphing into a full-blown company by 2018 that manufactured, wholesaled, and retailed CBD products. Dad never wanted to hear about it. He wanted nothing to do with "the reefer."

It didn't matter to him that the creams and tinctures I produced were made from hemp since he was unaware of the differences between that and the weed he knew from the '70s. He couldn't care less that the laws surrounding cannabis were rapidly changing all around. Even recreational use of weed had been legal for many years in Washington State, only 20 minutes away.

He was terrified of the plant. He had been traumatized and bullied by some "stoners" at his high school, which was only a few short miles from the Mexican-American border. It was only compounded by the media's portrayal and propaganda of the "war on drugs." Like so many others in his generation, he was brainwashed by the "reefer madness" narrative. I didn't see him even opening up to the idea that cannabis held therapeutic potential.

Let's get back to the story at hand.

I tricked him. He had just run out of the ointment that the VA had given him to ease the pain topically. I was curious about how well it was working for him since he went through it so quickly.

"Eh, it works a little better than IcyHot," he replied. "I have to use a lot, but it's better than nothing."

"On a scale from 1 to 10, how much better?" I asked.

"IcyHot? Took the pain from a 7 to a 5.5. Diclofenac [the stuff from the VA] took the pain levels to a 5," he muttered.

"Let me massage it a bit. I have some massage cream in my purse that I can use on you," I mentioned deceptively.

Within a couple of minutes of lightly massaging the cream into his shoulder, arm, wrist, and hand, you could see the tension lines on his face easing, and a deep sense of relief overcame him.

Yes, I had used one of my signature CBD creams on him. Yes, it was hemp and even legal in Idaho. No, it didn't get him high. Yes, he realized it wasn't just some ordinary massage cream I was using.

"What did you use?" he asked in wonder. "You barely worked on me, and it feels so much better!"

"Good," I said in a snarky tone.

"You know how I make CBD creams in my business? Well, now you know how they feel," I confessed.

He was shocked. I was worried he might flip out, as he's not exactly the cool-headed type. It was quiet for a while. To be fair, it's not like I got him high. I considered just grabbing my stuff and leaving his house before he decided to react. But then he said softly:

"Would it be okay if I told my VA doctor about this stuff? It's amazing."

"I would love that," I said. It was my turn to be shocked. I left the rest of the jar with him, and for a while, he told everyone he knew about my company, Herb 'N Oil.

He is now open to listening to the potential benefits that cannabis holds. He even calls me whenever there's a piece on the news about hemp or CBD, or even anything cannabis-related, really.

He finally recognized the thousands of hours I had put into researching this amazing plant. He understood the investment I made to get everything lab-tested, along with the effort I exerted to create clean, sustainable, and affordable wellness products. None of that would have happened had I not tricked him into it. Do I regret it? Not one bit. That being said, I don't endorse tricking people into using cannabis. He learned that not all cannabis gets you high.

***Myth #2: CBD will get me high.***
***Reality: Hemp CBD doesn't get you high; THC does.***

# CHAPTER FIVE

# MEDIA, POLITICS, AND MARIJUANA (OH MY!)

Why is "marijuana" a derogatory term?
What was "reefer madness"?
How did such a useful crop that held countless industrial and medical uses become so demonized?
Why do people either fully embrace cannabis or are completely revolted by it?

Let's take a look at a timeline of some major milestones and influences in both U.S. and Cannabis history. This is just a very brief overview, but it gives you a good idea of what a thriving industry it once was, what led to prohibition, as well as the fear that revolved around its usage just prior to its outlawing.

Starting in the 17th century, when our country was being established and decided to assert itself as an independent nation, domestically grown and manufactured hemp products were at the backbone of industry and agriculture in the colonies. European hemp was brought over and planted in fields to support the growth in the colonies. It was used for ropes, sails, clothing, fishing nets, paper products, and bedding.

This demand continued through the end of the Civil War.

Also, during this time, across the world, doctors, scientists, teachers, leaders, and researchers saw that cannabis was a common herb. It was used in various cultures for healing both physical ailments and mental health in spiritual rituals. It was also used as a means to slow aging and strengthen one's constitution.

In Asia, the Middle East, and North Africa, they were utilizing ALL parts of the plant. They ate it raw, blended it in drinks, smoked it, made tinctures with it, and created other blended herbal concoctions. People ate the seeds and steeped the roots, having recognized that even the parts that didn't produce psychoactive effects on the body were still valuable and beneficial.

Highly respected physicians from all over Europe were traveling along these trade routes to learn more about the remedies that were so common and popular among these cultures. After investigating and validating the legitimacy, many physicians and scientists wrote books about all the potential uses. They recorded their findings in case studies regarding the therapeutic use of cannabis for a wide variety of maladies. Some notable instances include *"Compleat Herbal"* (1645) and *"Edinburgh New Dispensatory"* (1794).

In the U.S., cannabis was utilized as a common household remedy. It was frequently found in the local apothecary, where an herbal clinician would compound the plant.

Oftentimes, the herbalist would blend it with other herbs for custom treatments based on the ailment.

Cannabis use continued through the late 19th century, in industrial hemp form and therapeutically as medicine. Recreational use of cannabis was frequently in the form of hashish and in hookahs. At this time, discreet hashish dens were speckled throughout every major American city. These dens provided a classy and luxurious social atmosphere where members of high society would come and partake in various forms of "psychoactive hemp" consumption—especially in baked goods. Those who partook capitalized on the ability to indulge without suffering hangover symptoms, giving them the freedom to maintain their affluent façade.

There was no stigma, no concerns about addiction, no violence, or other unsavory behaviors attached to usage. It was simply a growing number of people consuming and smoking (for a more brief but mild high). At this time, cannabis was used for both recreational and self-medicating purposes. As renowned doctors, clinicians, and scientists of the time explored the various preparations for this exciting herb, a young man by the name of Fitz High Ludlow wrote a related book. He took a more psychological and spiritual approach to the subject and called it *"The Hasheesh Eater"* (1857). His goal was to experience and document the knowledge, creativity, self-exploration, and insight gained through using higher and higher doses of hashish.

In 1860, the first official U.S. government medical study on cannabis was conducted. It provided a detailed examination of the array of medicinal uses for "psychoactive hemp" that had been proven effective by medical doctors. In fact, successful treatments for everything from P.M.S. (premenstrual syndrome), bronchitis, and rheumatism to venereal disease and migraines were just some of the medicinal uses. It became a go-to substance for pain relief. Even medical textbooks and journals had many specific types of pain for which the experts said it should be administered.

## Pharma Rises.

All these things competed with the emerging pharmaceutical industry. In 1852, the rise of mass-produced pharmaceuticals reduced the necessity of compounding apothecaries, coinciding with the founding of the American Pharmaceutical Association. Pharmaceutical companies employed research scientists to take the active ingredients of plant medicines and extract them in order to test, reproduce, or create (synthesize) them in laboratories.

*For example*:

*White willow bark contains salicin, which is and has been used as herbal medicine to treat pain, fevers, and joint inflammation.*

*The mechanism behind this is that the body converts salicin into salicylic acid, which reduces the production of the inflammation-causing chemical prostaglandin. Willow bark also contains flavonoids, which are plant compounds that have anti-inflammatory benefits.*

*Scientist Edward Stone, in the 1820s, used dried willow bark to extract salicin, then "purified" it in Germany. Shortly thereafter, a German chemist for Bayer, Felix Hoffman, was recruited to modify the isolated compound in order to improve its strength. He ended up synthesizing salicylic acid by acetylating it (the "A" in Aspirin). The "Spirin" came from the alternate source of salicin he used—the Spirea shrub. The standardized "Aspirin" was now the preferred substance over the more natural and readily available white willow bark.*

By this time, though, in the late 1800s, pharma companies were investing heavily in synthetic painkillers that could be patented and monopolized, like Aspirin in 1899. They could not only control the production and distribution of these patented medications but also the cost. Unfortunately, cannabis, being a low-cost and accessible substitution, threatened the control of medicine that the pharmaceutical industry was seeking.

In 1906, Theodore Roosevelt passed the Pure Food and Drug Act, which required regulation, labeling, and standardization of commercial medications, in lieu of compounding more personalized medicine. This law was developed with good intentions. It was designed to restrain abuse in the pharmaceutical industry by labeling substances with abuse potential as well as intoxicating qualities.

This also became the baseline for the current prescription system we have today. It gave the government and the pharmaceutical industry control over what drugs could be consumed. Although they still didn't see abuse potential, cannabis was wrapped into this legislation in order to take control of its usage. The federal government stipulated that cannabis could now only be imported for medical use.

Prior to this act, Sears sold heroin hypodermic kits. Cocaine was in Coca-Cola. Modern-day "illegal" drugs were sold as over-the-counter or mail-order commodities. This included alcohol, cannabis, cocaine, opiates, and others. This law would be a fast track to federal control over drugs—since, at this point, no drugs were deemed "illegal" yet.

In 1910, the Flexner Report was released. It was a study by Abraham Flexner, commissioned by the Carnegie Foundation. Flexner had no medical, healthcare, or scientific background. Regardless, this report evaluated medical education and called for reform in the medical schools and textbooks, and it was taught and implemented into what we know as "modern medicine." The Rockefeller Foundation gave "substantial funding" (estimated to be anywhere from $500 to $1 billion) in order to implement the recommendations. Start the American Medical Association (AMA) and ensure medical schools were aligned with the pharmaceutical and surgical model they were trying to establish, despite using only homeopathy for their personal medical care. This affected laws, policies, higher education, and the "capitalistic business" model that would end up setting the stage for mainstream medicine today (both good and bad).

- Stricter admission to medical schools with a curriculum based solely on scientific principles.

- The closure of many medical schools—the ones that taught herbal medicine, encouraged homeopathy, and allowed women and Black students—was targeted.
- Medical education shifted completely to a new model that taught research, pharmaceuticals, and surgery. The "biomedical model" excluded traditional (herbal and alternative) medicines that had been practiced for thousands of years with great success.
- Encouragement of medical schools to become associated with universities for research purposes. Research, engineering, and social sciences would now be exclusively taught in universities through scientific methods.

Shortly after, in 1914, the federal government decided it needed to make the distinction between medical and recreational drug use. This regulation would be spelled out by the Harrison Act, which made public, non-medical use of narcotics illegal. This was also the year that the media began its "fear" campaign against the Mexicans who were crossing the border into Texas and New Mexico. They called it *"loco weed," the* dangerous vice of the Hispanic population. This led to the city of El Paso, TX, passing an ordinance that banned the sale and possession of cannabis.

## Politics, media, racism, and greed.

Around 1910, after the Mexican Revolution, a few additional things happened that would lead to the demonization of cannabis. Political agendas, racism, and financial influence from the pharmaceutical and chemical industries now had the ability to control public perception through media outlets. These factors became the perfect storm that would eventually lead to cannabis prohibition in 1937.

Due to the Mexican Revolution and the thriving industry in the U.S., hundreds of thousands of Mexican migrants fled and crossed the southern border into the U.S., seeking safety and work.

Many of the immigrants also enjoyed the inexpensive, accessible, and relaxing effects of smoking "Mary Jane."

Also during this period, on the West Coast, a media mogul named William Randolph Hearst, out of San Francisco, had taken his father's failing publishing company and turned it around. With newspapers across the nation, his significant investment in the wood pulp-based paper milling industry made him a natural opponent to the less expensive and more durable hemp paper industry.

Along with wanting to rid the U.S. of the hemp paper industry, Hearst also had a personal vendetta against Mexicans. In 1916, Pancho Villa's *mota*[1] smoking troops occupied Hearst's 800,000-acre ranch and took over some of his cattle-grazing land in Chihuahua, MX. By connecting weed to the brown immigrants from the south, he was able to kill two birds with one stone. His widespread influence and political ties led to a collaboration with Harry Jacob Anslinger against cannabis.

The U.S. citizens knew hemp for its industrial purposes and also knew cannabis for its place in medicine—including the recreational aspect that was enjoyed as hashish. By calling cannabis *"marihuana"* in all the papers and media outlets, Hearst was doing both himself and Anslinger a favor by tricking the public into fearing this substance, brought over the border by the "migrants who were stealing American jobs."

Slowly, state legislatures started "believing" the false narratives that the media was providing regarding the "harms and crimes associated with immigrants smoking marihuana." It started with California in 1913, outlawing the herb in many western and southern states where minorities were more prevalent.

Anslinger was appointed by President Hoover to be the first commissioner of the Federal Bureau of Narcotics after being of great assistance to the alcohol prohibition efforts. He eventually became known as the "Godfather of America's War on Drugs." This appointment in 1930 was influenced by the U.S. Secretary of the Treasury at the time (who happened to be Anslinger's father-in-law), Andrew Mellon. Anslinger's backing from pharmaceutical companies and chemical industries laid a foundation that would support the desire to shut down the cannabis industry altogether.

When tax revenues plummeted during the Great Depression, Anslinger saw cannabis as the perfect scapegoat to bolster his personal résumé. Because of the popularity of "pot smoking" in jazz clubs, Anslinger portrayed marijuana as a dangerous substance that promoted sexual relations between the races and caused black men to lust after white women.

Hearst was also eager to sensationalize and even make up the harms of cannabis. Martin A. Lee writes in his book *Smoke Signals*, that "Hearst launched a smear campaign against Mexican migrants and their herb of choice. 'Murder Weed Found Up and Down Coast—Deadly Marihuana Dope Plant Ready for Harvest That Means Enslavement of California Children,' the *Los Angeles Examiner* screeched in 1933." He would print Anslinger's fabricated statistics on how crime was rampant among the jazz musicians (predominantly African American males), Mexicans, and Cuban immigrants.

His extreme prejudice against both the herb and the brown migrants of the time bled through the propaganda he was consistently spewing. It inspired Anslinger to take it a step further by traveling around the country to give speeches. At rallies, he warned of the dangers of cannabis in society, to churches, civic organizations, and anyone who would listen. These warnings were not only published in the newspapers but also in early films.

Anslinger pitched ideas that ended up becoming a couple of low-budget films. One film was funded by distilleries, a natural competitor to the cannabis industry during Prohibition. The other was funded by a church group. These films aimed to stir up enough outrage that cannabis would be outlawed. The titles, *Marihuana!* (1935) and *Tell Your Children* (1936) preyed on the worst fears of the time and incorporated the racial divide that both Hearst and Anslinger were trying to associate with cannabis usage. The first film, *Marihuana!* was about a young woman who smokes marijuana, which led her down a rabbit hole of crime, pregnancy, and immorality. The second film, *Tell Your Children*, (which ended up being renamed *"Reefer Madness"*), was a highly exaggerated cautionary tale of teenagers who get lured into marijuana use, which resulted in insanity, addiction, promiscuity, and murder.

Between Hearst and Anslinger's agendas, they were able to steer the public narrative—creating fear, divisiveness, and confusion. This all culminated in the "Marihuana Tax Act of 1937," which outlawed cannabis on a federal level.

# US Cannabis History

## 17th Century

*Hemp agriculture was encouraged by the government for the production of rope, sails and clothing. It was even produced as a durable paper for important documents. In 1776, the Declaration of Independence was signed...on hemp paper. G. Washington says "Sow it everywhere!"*

↓

## 1865–1910

*Up until the end of the Civil War, domestic production flourished. The end of the Civil War opened the door to importing goods that ended up replacing hemp for many things. It was also during this time that cannabis was really being utilized as medicine and was sold openly in apothecaries & pharmacies- often as tinctures for everything from rheumatism to seizures.*

↓

## 1910–1935

*Post Mexican Revolution, mexican immigrants, along with recreational use of cannabis, flooded the US. Going into the Depression Era, unemployment had skyrocketed. William Randolf Hearst (publishing mogul) felt threated the the hemp industry would replace his paper-producing companies. He popularized an "anti-cannabis crusade" and stigmatized "marijuana" use by associating brown migrants to job scarcity & "drug use" in order to eliminate hemp paper as a competing product.*

### 1934-1937

*Director of the Federal Bureau of Narcotics (FBN) Harry Jacob Anslinger jumped on board with William Randolf Hearst's media campaign against cannabis. The FBN was hurting for revenue and Anslinger used the opportunity to demonize cannabis for monetary gain. By calling it marijuana, they tricked the public into thinking it was different than the Hemp and Cannabis that had been part of their daily life as a medicine & commodity.*

### 1937-1969

*By 1937, marijuana was officially criminalized in the US. The films Marijuana! & Reefer Madness were a key part of the propaganda leading to cannabis prohibition. They created the narrative that Mexicans & African Americans, while under the influence of marijuana, would "lust after" white women- leading to "degradation & orgies." In order to "support" the new ban, statistics were fabricated- citing use amongst minorities & the relationship to increase in crime.*

### 1970s-1996

*In 1970, still calling it "marijuana" the Controlled substance act classifies it as a Schedule 1 drug along with heroin & LSD...saying it has "relatively the highest abuse potential with no accepted medical use " Yet Fentanyl and Cocaine are in a more lenient category. By now, cannabis use was a sign of rebellion. Nixon launched the "war on drugs" in 1971. In 1973 he founded the DEA and Oregon decriminalizes cannabis. The Reagan era launched the DARE campaign.*

### 1996-2012

*A turning point in US cannabis law, California becomes the 1st state to legalize medical cannabis which starts a trend. By 2016, a majority of states now have some form of a medical cannabis law or program. Average plant potency has significantly risen over this period of time from 4% THC in 1995 to 12% in 2014 while the avg. CBD potency has fallen from .28% in 2001- <.15% in 2014.*

### 2012-2025

*Washington and Colorado become the first states to legalize recreational cannabis. By the time of this writing, in early 2025, Ohio becomes the 24th state (+Washington DC) to legalize recreational cannabis. This year, cannabis is FINALLY supposed to be rescheduled as a Schedule III drug or become federally decriminalized over 70% of the population supports this. 4 states (Idaho, Wyoming, Kansas & South Carolina) remain without any legal THC use- not even less than .3% in hemp products.*

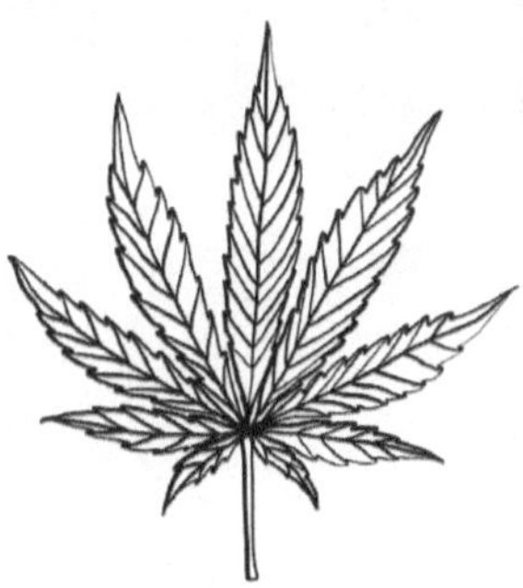

For a more complete history on cannabis, *Smoke Signals* by Martin A. Lee is a fantastic comprehensive resource.

# PART II

# CANNASCIENCE AND YOU

## BOTANY, PLANT MAGIC AND MODERN PRODUCT DEVELOPMENT

# CHAPTER SIX

# PLANT ANATOMY

The history, the laws, and the stigma tell their own tale, but as you can see by now, there must be something special about this plant in order for it to stir up so much emotion, controversy, and attention. Prior to the U.S. being formed and governed, it had been a consistent part of worldwide history for millennia. This plant was steeped in cultural rituals, integrated into ancient wellness practices, and traded as a valuable commodity. Shared between neighbors, it brought together a sense of camaraderie among varying races, religions, and socioeconomic statuses. To understand more about cannabis's intrinsic value, let's get to the "root" of the issue and learn about the plant itself—starting with its anatomy.

You now understand that the seeds and the roots of cannabis plants contain no CBD (or THC for that matter), but what parts of the plant do, and where is it most abundant? You may also be wondering where hemp seeds come from and how many parts of the plant are usable. These facts are all important to know for those looking to enter the industry and for home growers alike.

We'll start by highlighting the basic plant growth cycle. Cannabis is considered dioecious since it has male and female parts on separate plants, so we will go over plant parts and their roles in development before we cover "gendered" parts, lab breeding, and natural reproduction.

In a world of a dominant patriarchy, the matriarchy "rules" when it comes to the therapeutic and recreational use of our favorite plant. Don't dismiss the importance of the males, though; they play an important, but more often overlooked, role in this industry.

## Basic Cannabis Parts

### ~From Bottom to Top~

### Roots

The basic function of the roots is to anchor the plant and absorb water and nutrients for optimal growth. Cannabis roots tend to grow more horizontally rather than deeply, as the depth is influenced by the quality and moisture of the soil. In ideal conditions, the roots could extend 2 to 3 feet deep in well-aerated substrate.

Since cannabis is a bioaccumulator, it absorbs nutrients, minerals, and even chemicals from whatever medium it is planted in. This means that whatever touches the roots will eventually be passed on to the consumer. This makes the soil, water, and nutrient quality EXTREMELY important when it comes to a clean and healthy end product.

It is important for growers to know and understand their soil's health prior to planting. If a farmer is planting a hemp crop on a farm that previously used pesticides, the residual chemicals from the pesticides may still be in the soil. Even if it was many years ago, the pesticides would be absorbed by the hemp plant and test "dirty" for pesticides during testing and harvest.

On the other end of that spectrum, industrial hemp has been used many times throughout history to "clean up" contaminants from the soil—a technique known as *phytoremediation*. Nicknamed a "mop crop," hemp has been used worldwide to destroy nematodes and other pests, remediate (or remove) radiation from nuclear sites such as Chernobyl, restore soil near sewage treatment plants, and even rehabilitate the soil in areas affected by acid rain.

Since the soil becomes depleted after each growth cycle, it is important to replenish the organic content either through regenerative farming, composting, adding new soil, and/or implementing additional nutrients and fertilizers. If you grow hydroponically, this is not a concern, as you would already be adding these to your water.

**Stalk**

Both male and female plants have a strong, hollow center stem called the "stalk." This part of the plant is responsible for creating a supportive structure, as well as for the transportation of water, nutrients, and sugars.

The stalk is the part of the plant harvested for fiber in industrial hemp applications. When grown for fiber, hemp plants are planted close together outdoors and can reach up to 20 ft tall. When grown for industrial purposes, one of the challenges that farmers face is the harvesting of the *biomass* due to the length and strength of the hemp fiber. Biomass is considered the non-flower parts of the plant. For larger crops (multiple acres), modifications are often needed on modern combines in order to handle the specific demands of industrial hemp farming. For smaller crops, a simple sickle can be used.

In general, the plants tend to be tall and slender (planted closer together for seed and fiber production) or short and thicker, allowing space to bloom. Flower/bud production requires a thicker stalk to support the weight, regardless of the intention to produce THC or CBD.

When growing for recreational or medical purposes, it is important to provide plenty of room for air circulation—both outdoors and indoors. Having the stressor of moving air, either naturally or artificially, is important to give the plant a chance to develop a stronger, thicker stalk to support heavy buds. Some growers say that a 1-inch diameter stalk equals a 1-pound yield, a 2-inch stalk equals a 2-pound yield, and so on. It is important to note that there are very few cannabinoids, including THC and CBD, in the stalks of cannabis plants. Unfortunately, due to current laws, the biomass in recreational and medicinal plants is supposed to be discarded despite the plethora of uses and nutritional value it still holds.

### Fan Leaves

The large, beautiful leaves that are commonly known to identify a cannabis plant are called "fan leaves" and hold the huge responsibility of *photosynthesis*, or converting sunlight, water, and carbon dioxide into energy and oxygen.

Because this special plant has such an incredible ability to sequester carbon dioxide from the atmosphere, there has been much speculation and ongoing studies about the amount of CO2 that can be pulled from the air and converted into oxygen. A 2022 study done by Hudson Carbon found that 1 acre of cannabis plants can absorb over 7 tons of carbon dioxide from the air and store up to 3 of those tons, with less water usage than most other crops. This is more than double the amount of CO2 that trees sequester, with significantly fewer water needs.

Ultimately, fan leaves are responsible for the growth of the entire plant. The larger and healthier these leaves are, the better their ability to produce the beneficial chemicals within the plant.

Visually, these iconic leaves are recognized worldwide, across all cultures. The colors, though typically green, can range from brownish-red to yellow to blue, purple, or even black, based on their strain and/or pH levels. The 5 to 9 fingers or points of the leaf can be long and slender (sativa-dominant types) or shorter and thicker (indica-dominant varieties) and have serrated edges and a delicate stem.

Although the fan leaves are often removed when cultivating

cannabis for medicinal use, the ones closer to the flower can contain trichomes, which are often used in recipes made with trim.

### Nodes

They are found where the lateral branch meets the stem and are a site for new growth, also known as growth tips. Nodes are important for identifying the sex of the plant. They look different on males and females and are sometimes referred to as "preflowers," even though it is only the females that produce the flowers/buds. Nodes consist of three parts: the reproductive organs, growth tips, and stipules.

### Stipules

These small leaf appendages, located at future bud sites, are short-lived. Their speculated purpose is to protect the forming reproductive organs.

## Male Cannabis Parts

### Nodes - male

Male plants carry a small, bell-shaped cluster found in the "armpit," between the stem and the lateral branches. They are typically in opposite pairs. Basically, they are the testicles of the male plant. The male nodes produce pollen sacs that have a more bulbous appearance and appear in the first three to five weeks of sprouting (in the late vegetative state).

## Pollen Sacs

Only the male node sites form pollen sacs. These sacs hang off the node site, producing and holding the pollen. Once these pollen sacs burst open, they fertilize the female plant through wind pollination, which occurs about four to five weeks into the plant's flowering stage.

*Cannabis pollen can travel naturally in the wind up to 30 miles! This disproves the common misconception that the cannabis plant relies on pollinators such as bees, butterflies, various other insects, and birds.*

Since the pollen is easily picked up and carried by the wind, it can be a challenge for outdoor farms to protect themselves from cross-pollination with neighboring fields of different cultivars. Medical and recreational cannabis farmers, as well as hemp farmers, want to avoid this as much as possible. This can destroy their ability to produce their intended end product on both sides.

Ex. #1: Hemp males → Cannabis females = Cannabis females with seeds = lower cannabinoid content, which produces a lower quality of product for them to sell or use.

Ex. #2: Cannabis males —> Hemp females = "hot crop" = will no longer qualify as "hemp" due to an overproduction of THC. The farmer must destroy the entire crop if required testing goes above the threshold. No viable product is left, as the entire field must be destroyed.

## Female Cannabis Parts

The female cannabis plant is the most sought-after sex due to the flowers and the concentration of therapeutic and potentially intoxicating chemicals that it contains. The main chemicals that create these effects are called cannabinoids and terpenes. THC and CBD are the most well-known cannabinoids. Although there are over 100 different cannabinoids that have been identified in the cannabis plant, which interact with our body's endocannabinoid system, THC and CBD remain the most popular, abundant, and well-studied. We will cover these in detail in later chapters, as they will have a significant effect on the user. We will discover that each cannabinoid and terpene has its own set of special "superpowers."

First, we will cover the flower itself and the parts that make it up, as well as how it reproduces. This will include HOW and WHY it produces the compounds for which this plant is so popular.

### Nodes - female

It is important to be able to distinguish a female plant from a male plant as early as possible in the plant's vegetative state. When the nodes are first forming on a female plant, they produce pistils that are longer and narrower than the male reproductive parts. These female organs are upward-facing and come to a point at the top, where they have translucent, hair-like stigmas that sprout out of the top of each female node. Each node will develop into a flower. The flower is where most of the magic happens and is likely the part that you have used if you have ever partaken in cannabis consumption of any sort.

### Flower

The flower typically is the "heroine" of our story here, as this is where the therapeutic compounds, such as CBD, are concentrated. The cannabis "flower" usually refers to the clusters of flowers found throughout the cannabis plant. The parts of a flower include the reproductive organ called the pistil.

### Cola

The cola is the main flower part commonly known as the "bud" (or just bud). It is a dense grouping of flowers. Anywhere from 30 to 150 small flowers are naturally found at the top of the female plant and at the ends of some stems. Smaller colas can also develop in the nodes, and the plant can be trimmed in a way to force more colas to form for a larger yield.

Each individual flower has the ability to carry a seed. This means that each cola can potentially carry anywhere from 30 to 150 seeds (although for therapeutic or recreational use, you want to avoid fertilization or going to seed, as that will lower the efficacy). The number of colas per plant can range greatly. I have seen anywhere from 3 large colas to 32 small to medium-sized colas per plant!

Some growers prefer a few large plants with a lot of smaller colas, whereas others have many plants with fewer large colas. It really can vary based on your goals, legal limitations, variety of plant, growth medium, space available, and method of growing. Fewer but larger colas allow for more air circulation and reduce the chance of mold. However, some argue that smaller buds have a more concentrated, potent effect. Every experienced grower has their own style of growing and will often adapt based on the individual plant's needs.

### Sugar leaves

Sugar leaves are tiny versions of fan leaves that grow in between the flowers and "cup" the buds. They are found throughout the cola and have many trichomes.

### Pistils

The pistil refers to the entire female reproductive organ, which forms part of the flower; it is sometimes known as the ovary of the plant. Pistils consist of a single ovule, which is encapsulated by many bracts (which make up the bulk of the bud), two stigmas, and two styles.

### Stigmas

These fuzzy-looking stigmas often grow to be ¼ to ½ inch long and are sticky, to easily catch the pollen that blows by in the wind. In controlled environments, this is where the breeder will apply the pollen during the flowering stage—ideally, 14 to 21 days in. While these are often called "pistils" in the cannabis community, this is incorrect. The stigmas (usually two) are attached to an ovule within a single pistil by a style.

**Style**

The style is a sturdy structure that attaches the stigma to the ovule. It acts as a conduit for pollen to travel down the stigma in order to fertilize the ovule.

**Ovule**

This is the prospective seed within a single flower. It can only form into a seed if fertilized by the pollen from a male plant. There are two stigmas that are attached to the single ovule by styles.

**Bracts**

Within the flower you will find tiny leaves that surround the reproductive cells of the female, called bracts. They are small, pear-shaped leaves that enclose the ovule, forming the outer portion of the flower—in essence, the "petals" of the cannabis bud. They are covered in resin glands (a.k.a. trichomes), which are rich in cannabinoids and terpenes.

**Trichomes**

Trichomes are easy to recognize on a cannabis plant. They essentially make it sparkle. These tiny crystalline structures form a sticky layer that covers the flowers, sugar leaves, bracts, and, to a lesser extent, the fan leaves. They are so important in producing the therapeutic compounds for which this plant is famous—the resin that contains flavonoids, cannabinoids, and terpenes.

Unpollinated flowers have more trichomes, which results in higher potency. The trichomes serve the purpose of protecting the plant from insects and predators, and even from the sun while it is growing.

**Seeds**

Seeds are created when male plants pollinate and fertilize the female pistils. They are typically undesirable for recreational and therapeutic growers in the industry, UNLESS they are breeding for new genetics or to improve the quality of a strain or variety.

It is a very common practice for both home and commercial growers to either buy feminized seeds or start from a clone of the female plant in order to ensure a female for flowering.

Seeds typically germinate in 3 to 7 days. When growing a young seedling, be aware that when the young female plant endures too many external stressors, it can potentially develop pollen sacs (called rhodelization), thus making it a hermaphrodite. These are best kept away from females if you are growing for maximum cannabinoid content.

Aside from producing new plants, hemp seeds are pressed to produce hemp seed oil or consumed whole for their incredible nutrient content.

* * *

These plant parts hold incredible medicinal and therapeutic value, especially, as we discussed previously, in the flower. All forms of cannabis have cannabinoids, terpenes, and other constituents that are widely recognized as having healing powers. There are many cultivars (phenotypes and combinations of these properties—commonly known as *strains*). Resources such as the app *Leafly* have a comprehensive library dedicated to describing individual strains of cannabis. Therefore, I decided to focus less on individual strains and more on the constituents (chemical makeup) most commonly valued in the cannabis plant. This is based on our modern understanding of how they interact with the body and the effects or benefits we can obtain from their unique composition.

# CHAPTER SEVEN

# CANNABIS CHEMICALS THAT CAN ROCK YOUR WORLD

There are currently 779 recognized cultivars (a.k.a. strains) that offer different combinations of cannabinoids, terpenes, and flavonoid profiles—more on what these are in just a bit. Each cultivar has its own unique benefits.

This is important to remember when trying any form of cannabis as the results can vary greatly from plant to plant. Remember "energetic creativity" vs. "couch lock" Some may describe this as a sativa vs. indica, but it truly is more complex than that since a majority of the products out on the market today are some form of a hybrid.

Traditionally, "sativas" were considered more energizing, with a "head high," whereas "indicas" tended to be more sedating, with a "body high." Nowadays, we have learned that it isn't that straightforward. Even more, hemp (which will not get you high) can be found in more energizing cultivars as well as relaxing cultivars.

Research has taught us that it is the terpenes, often in combination with both major and minor cannabinoids, that dictate how the body reacts to these specific plant chemicals.

## What are cannabinoids?

Cannabinoids are chemical compounds made either by the cannabis plant (phytocannabinoid) or by the human body (endocannabinoid). Both types of cannabinoids make an impact throughout the body in various ways. In this chapter, we will discuss many of the major and minor phytocannabinoids that are found in the plants. Each cannabinoid has its own unique chemical structure and interaction within the body.

We will just refer to phytocannabinoids—the ones found in plants—as cannabinoids from here on out. When we start talking about our body's naturally produced cannabinoids, we will refer to those as *endo*cannabinoids or by their specific chemical names.

There are over 100 different cannabinoids found in the cannabis plant. We will only cover the ones most abundant in the plant, the ones being clinically researched that you can currently (as of 2025) find advertised on the market in some form.

Keep in mind, when we talk about the effects of a phytocannabinoid, we are referring to only the effect of the specific cannabinoid. We are not referring to the way in which it interacts with other plant chemicals, such as terpenes, which enhance the effect or give it some variations. When used in its whole plant form, there are MANY (hundreds) of natural plant chemicals in cannabis that produce the therapeutic effect, which changes from strain to strain. For clarity, when we discuss the effect of THC, it is ONLY THC, not in combination with CBD (another major cannabinoid), or not when myrcene (a terpene) is also present.

When referring to THC, CBD and other cannabinoids, I will only be talking about naturally found cannabinoids, not lab-created or synthetic cannabinoids. Those will be discussed in a later chapter since they do not always have the same therapeutic value, potential side effects, and uses.

*A note about clinical research:*

*We (the general public, businesses, the medical community and patients) rely on clinical research to guide us in the dosing and usage of products and the development of supplements and pharmaceuticals.*

*It is important to note that no two people will react exactly the same to the same substance. It is also imperative to note that these studies often rely on volunteers and participants from the community who may or may not have a variety of underlying conditions (which may or may not be diagnosed and/or disclosed during the application process). The research groups may have a tendency to be predominantly one gender, race, socioeconomic class, or age.*

*The final note I feel is important is being aware of WHAT kind of product is being tested. Is the same strain/variety being used throughout the entire study and for every participant? What cannabinoids and terpenes are present that may impact results? What is the method of consumption (smoking, vaping, edibles, etc.), and how much is being used for these trials? There are some solid trials out there that define all these parameters, but MANY do not.*

*Some of the research may be sponsored by a particular brand, pharmaceutical company, or university. It can be helpful to know and understand the goal of the study. Are researchers looking to utilize it to treat a specific disease? Are they determining the safety of a product at high doses? Are they identifying potential interactions with other medications? There are a host of potential goals and queries that may be present for a single study. It is also helpful to know the source of the products being used for research. I have heard of everything from participants supplying their own to synthetically produced or lab-created products, all the way to government-issued or grown cannabis.*

We will cover WHY these things are important to know and how each of these factors play a huge role, in the outcome when used medicinally and therapeutically.

## Major Cannabinoids: THC and CBD

Major cannabinoids are found in greater abundance in the cannabis plant. They are well known, have been widely studied, and are heavily marketed. The commonly known major cannabinoids are CBD and THC, and they are also the cannabinoids found in the highest quantities within the cannabis plant. Both CBD and THC have different effects on the human body, and their effects can also vary in individuals, which we will explore further when we discuss the endocannabinoid system.

Many products have BOTH THC and CBD in varying amounts when in their natural form, as well as other minor cannabinoids, terpenes, waxes, flavonoids, chlorophyll, and other fats and nutrients. Let's dive into these a bit.

Cannabidiol (CBD) is found predominantly in hemp and medical cannabis. CBD is widely used for a multitude of conditions but is mostly known for its anti-inflammatory, anti-anxiety, anti-seizure, and anticancer properties. It is non-intoxicating and has powerful antioxidant and antibacterial properties. (See more benefits in Chapters 18 and 19.)

Delta 9-Tetrahydrocannabinol (THC)- found in the highest concentrations in recreational and medical cannabis. Negligible amounts (.3%) are found in hemp. THC has intoxicating effects that can provide pain relief, muscle relaxation, reduce intraocular eye pressure (glaucoma), anti-nausea effects, and can induce appetite.

The legality of cannabis products is dependent on the amounts of THC in each product. THC can also enhance the effect of other cannabinoids, a phenomenon known as the "entourage effect."

Even though these cannabinoids are found in abundance naturally in cannabis plants, they can still be synthesized or created in a lab. Quite often, these lab-created versions are utilized for research or to create a pharmaceutical "standardized" product. (More on this in Chapter 19.)

## Minor or "rare" cannabinoids are still important!

CBC and CBG, along with the acidic forms of CBD and THC (called CBDa and THCa, respectively), are the next highest quantities of cannabinoids naturally found within the plant. Many cannabinoids have an acidic form. This is how they are naturally found in the plant before they undergo decarboxylation—the process of applying heat to remove the carboxyl group. This process is often done by smoking, vaping, cooking, or baking the bud. In commercial production, this is also done during either processing or manufacturing finished products (such as edibles) that will not be smoked or vaped.

Previously, this was thought to "activate" the product since it would convert THCA → THC. THCA doesn't get you high, but once that bond is broken and it converts to its neutral form, THC, it does. Ironically, THCA is actually more potent than they once thought. THCA is now being researched for its own unique therapeutic benefits, even though it is non-intoxicating in this form.

On the next page, I have included a "clock" of 10 of the most commonly found, naturally occurring "rare" cannabinoids. It includes any known benefits, with the most abundant cannabinoid, Delta-9 THC, at the 12 o'clock position and CBD at the 6 o'clock position. The corresponding numbers denote known benefits and properties associated with each cannabinoid. Minor cannabinoids are only found in trace amounts, but don't count them out, since many therapeutic drugs have been found in plants from only minuscule amounts of a substance.

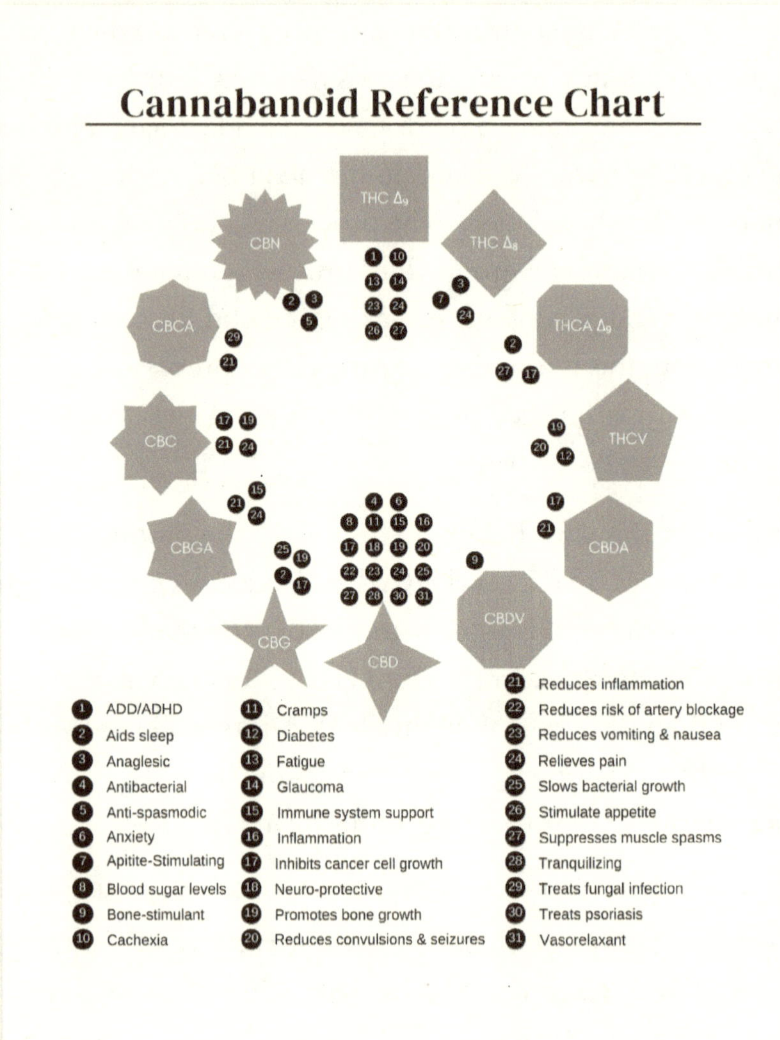

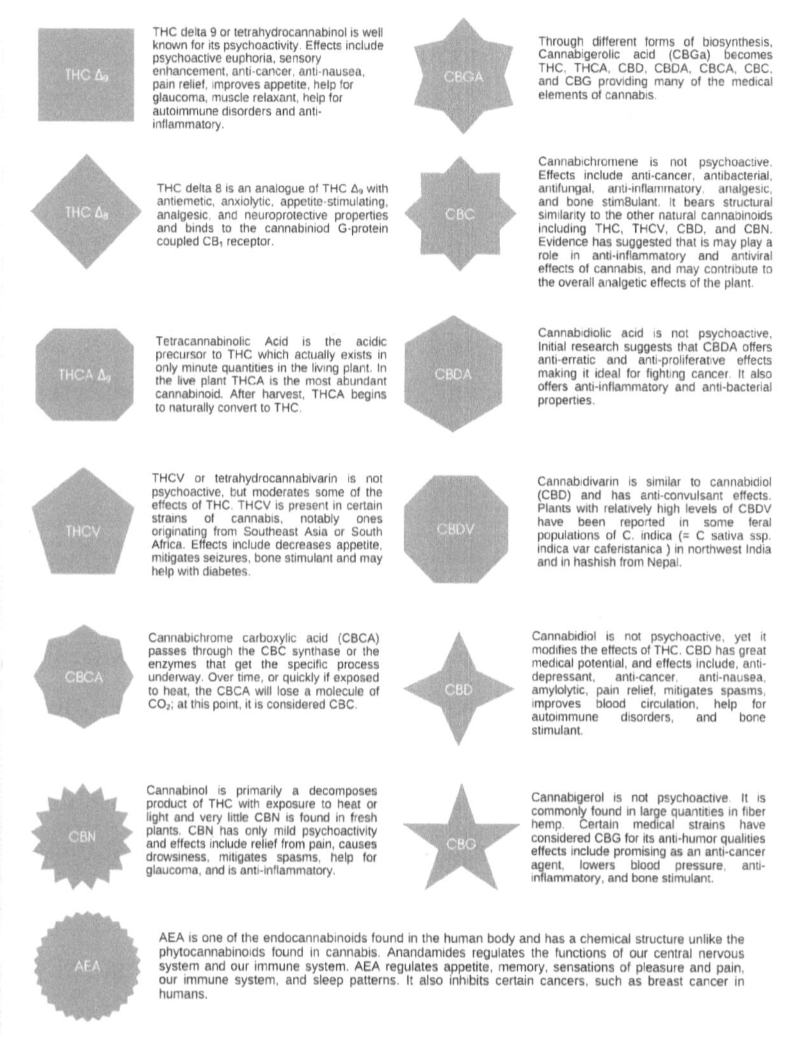


You may wonder why HHC, HXC, THC-P, and others aren't on this list. It is because these are considered "lab-created" cannabinoids. They are not found naturally occurring but are created by altering natural cannabinoids or by "growing them" from yeasts, esters, and other chemicals within a lab setting. Some of the natural minor cannabinoids can be lab-created as well. These synthetic cannabinoids will be discussed in Part 3.

## Terpenes

Terpenes are aromatic compounds found in plants that contribute to the distinct smells and flavors of different strains. They are what give lemons their fragrant scent and lavender its relaxing effect. There are around 250 different terpenes found in the cannabis plant. Each one contributes to a unique aroma and potential effects.

On a biological level, their purpose is to defend the plant against herbivores (everything from insects to deer), act as hormones, and can also be responsible for cellular signaling. According to industrial hemp farms, researchers commonly categorize them into 4 broad flavor profiles: sweet, sour, spicy, or bitter. They also emphasize that the terpenes need to be heated to a certain point in order to transform them into an "activated form."

A "high" percentage of terpenes in any given cannabis strain would be over 2%, but some can have as much as 5-10% terpene content. If you walk into a dispensary and are able to "smell sample" the buds, you may notice similar scents between them; however, some may have stronger scent profiles. Some may smell more musty, fruity, grassy, earthy, woodsy, or like honey.

The six most common cannabis (both hemp and THC-heavy) terpenes, their activation temperature, and their most prominent benefits in cannabis are:

- Myrcene—sedates, increases appetite (332°F).
- Linalool—relieves stress and insomnia (388°F).
- A-Pinene provides memory retention and alertness (311°F).
- Limonene: anti-depressant effects, anti-anxiety (348°F)
- Humulene acts like an appetite suppressant and mood booster (222°F).
- Caryophyllene reduces pain and muscle spasms (266°F).

Since every terpene has its own scent, properties, and therapeutic effect, I am sure you can imagine the number of combinations of terpenes in various strains. Some are polar opposites. These are important to be aware of if you are a medical marijuana patient or using hemp products therapeutically. One strain may help an ailment, while another may aggravate it.

*For example:*

*Myrcene has an earthy, musky aroma and is known to have relaxing and sedative effects. It is also an appetite stimulant.*

*Humulene has an earthy aroma, with woody and spicy notes. Humulene has more energizing and uplifting qualities and tends to be an appetite suppressant. Within clinical applications, you wouldn't want to give a recovering anorexic a strain high in humulene, but one high in myrcene could be beneficial for weight gain and to restore an appetite.*

## Flavonoids, lipids, and waxes.

Whole plant usage will allow the user to utilize nutrients that get filtered out or damaged during processing. Nutritionally speaking, the ideal way to consume a cannabis plant would be raw. This would be akin to eating fresh veggies. No nutrients are lost, depleted, or destroyed. Canna juice, anyone?

The flavonoids, lipids, waxes, and more contain antioxidants, minerals, and vitamins. They also promote cellular health. Flavonoids specifically tend to have anti-inflammatory, antioxidant, anti-cancer, and neuroprotective properties, which are all supportive of overall well-being. While some flavonoids have been demonized for their phytoestrogenic properties (more on that in Chapter 16), the ones found in the raw cannabis plant do not impact hormonal balance in a significant way. The lipids and waxes are important for cell structure and functioning, as well as for optimizing nutrient absorption and promoting cardiovascular health.

If you grow your own cannabis products, don't let those leaves go to waste! Toss them in soups or salads, add them to your sandwich, juice them, dry them, and steep them with your favorite tea![2]

* * *

With all of these incredible benefits and health-supporting attributes, it is no wonder the pharmaceutical industry felt threatened by this incredibly versatile plant! While cannabis can be consumed in many traditional ways still, it is worth noting that modern processing and extraction methods have taken the cannabis industry to a whole new level. These methods allow terpenes to be extracted or even added, cannabinoid concentrations to be manipulated, and cannabis to be infused in almost any kind of product. (We'll discuss this more in the next chapter.)

## CHAPTER EIGHT

# HOW ARE CANNABIS PRODUCTS MADE?

Do you think that the people who are getting healthy, with optimal results from adding cannabis products to their lifestyle, are buying CBD from a gas station? What about taking gummies filled with artificial colors and laden with heavy metals? Or taking tinctures that were manufactured in China, which contain pesticides and molds in the distillates used for formulation?

Although the demand for quality products has never diminished, recent years have seen a new generation of users and consumers seeking specific niche products in the regulated U.S. markets. The open availability in recreational cannabis states has led to a true buyer's market. Brands are vying for public approval and customers with brightly colored edibles packaging, "craft" bud bars, bougie lounge-style dispensaries, flower "release" parties, and marketing promos that range from "happy hour" deals to branded merch.

This type of competition leads to larger companies cutting corners and sacrificing quality for quantity in order to cash in on more lucrative profit margins. Yep, we are in the midst of "cannabis capitalism." The floodgates are open.

For too many people, the extraction and manufacturing process doesn't matter. However, there are smart people out there who tend to obsess about these details—either because they are curious about how it goes from seed to sale (maybe due to personal interest or professional development) or because their bodies are sensitive to the various constituents and additives (like me). These variants matter in the efficacy of products and how the body reacts to them—both natural and manufactured. This is just a brief overview of the most common processes, transforming a beautiful plant into a dried smokable bud and potentially a liquid extract (to be made into an oil, tincture, vape cartridge, concentrate, topical, or edible). The process is the same for all types of cannabis (hemp, recreational, or medical), but the differences lie in the goals of the person consuming or the company selling the end product.

Below are two examples of ways taking cannabis can unintentionally go wrong in a legal, seemingly safe setting. This is not to discourage usage but to encourage awareness. It will hopefully also inspire you to continue to learn about the things you put in your body. The goal is to have a safe, positive, and healthy relationship with cannabis.

*Example #1*

*An amazing initial flower strain, when combined with crappy ingredients in an edible—let's take high fructose corn syrup and red #3 as examples—can make a person feel sick, agitated, and anxious, while that same flower strain, in a dry herb vaporizer, can create a feeling of blissful, calm contentment.*

*The above scenario can happen anywhere—at a house party with homemade edibles (e.g., red velvet cake mix brownies) or at a reputable dispensary that is fully regulated, tested, and taxed.*

*Example #2*

*Now, let's take Hemp CBD tinctures, as an example. Two brands are sitting on the shelf side-by-side. They have the same dosage strength, same type (full spectrum- less than .3% THC), and same ingredients: Full spectrum hemp extract, hemp seed oil. You would think that these 2 products would "work the same" for the same person, but that isn't always the case.*

*The analysis:*

*Given additional information that the general public may or may not be aware of, one brand provides 3rd party testing, while one does not. There is a good chance that the one that provides the testing is more expensive than the one without, but not always.*

*One product may work wonderfully, reducing the customer's inflammation levels and helping them sleep better at night. However, the other one, seemingly the same, causes nausea, headache and restlessness at night. It is possible that the one bottle that went untested was labeled properly, with all the things in it, including the less than .3% THC limit for hemp products. What also could have happened is that the process of extraction used, left residual solvents behind, making the user sick, turning them away from the potential that a "clean" CBD product could hold for them. The tested product would have shown this in its lab results. Ideally, the person responsible for sourcing these products would be aware of these testing results, prior to selling the merchandise to the retailer or customers. In the current state of the industry, though, it is "buyer beware."*

These types of scenarios are, unfortunately, extremely common in this industry. When product education is lacking and monetary gain is prioritized over public health and safety, the industry suffers as a whole. I have heard COUNTLESS times that CBD didn't work for someone, and that a hemp product retailer didn't realize that lab testing was a "thing." I have also heard accounts of customers having no clue or guidance on potential medication interactions, dosage, or even knowing what kind (full spectrum, broad spectrum, or isolate) of internal use product would help them reach their goals. I have even heard a lot of frustration over these things on the recreational side of the industry. Lack of training and education in every arm of the industry bleeds through and affects consumers.

Methods, ingredients, and quality matter.

Regulated medical and recreational cannabis markets that allow retail sales of products have guidelines for growing, processing (if any), manufacturing (if any), testing, and labeling. Strictly adhering to these guidelines is expensive—from the licenses, permits, auditors, inspectors, labs, and additional state fees to the actual costs of growing, processing, and/or manufacturing. The hemp CBD market does not have these same guidelines and regulations for the most part since it is not under the FDA's purview (as of 2025);

therefore, it is not subject to many, if any, requirements from wholesalers and retailers.

If you live in an area where you are fortunate enough to grow your own plants, what an opportunity to have control over these things! You may choose to do very minimal interventions with your plant medicine. As we learned in Chapter 6, "Plant Anatomy," under the section labeled "Roots," even if you grow your own medicine, the soil or other growing medium, water quality, and any added nutrients are important because they aid in the final product. You can choose to grow an organic product. You have the right and responsibility to test the soil (or other growing medium) and water for contaminants such as chlorine, molds, mildews, heavy metals, and so on.

When you are purchasing products from a dispensary, you are relying on the grower, processor, or manufacturer to do all the legwork to provide the retailer, and ultimately the customer, with a product that is clean, safe, and tested. Unfortunately, there is not the same type of reliability when you are purchasing CBD products in most cases. Although in some states, hemp CBD is sold and regulated under the same or similar umbrella as recreational cannabis, this is the exception, not the rule at the moment. Due to the unregulated hemp and CBD market, many stores only need to have a resale/wholesaling permit to buy and sell CBD products. Depending on where these products are sourced, manufactured, or formulated, the regulations may be nonexistent.

There are many touchpoints along the supply chain where a product can potentially fall short in terms of both quality and safety. I will just briefly touch on the typical supply chain and ways that each leg of the industry can ensure a reliable product that is safe, effective, legal, and high-quality for the customer.

## Growers/Farmers

It is hard work and a LOT of trial and error when it comes to growing ANY plants, but when you are taking a product to market for public consumption, you want to get the most bang for your buck. This begins with research, training, and a lot of prep work.

Quality products, whether grown from seed or clone, indoors or outdoors, will need a high-quality, tested growth medium, nutrients, and water. Questions you might ask are: Is the irrigation water full of lead? Has your soil been tested for pesticides? Are your nutrients optimal for the growing stage your plant is in? Is your crop protected from cross-pollination or overspray from neighboring farms? Is your humidity and air circulation optimal to prevent pests, mold, and mildew if you are growing indoors or in a greenhouse? Testing is essential. Test the soil and water to find out what minerals are present or lacking. Learn about the microbes that are present. Test for cannabinoid content. Once the product has been harvested and dried, test again before processing—1st party testing. This is now considered biomass.

At this point, it goes through one or more of the following steps:

1. The biomass is trimmed and packaged as flower/bud or processed in-house, if the law allows.
2. It's shipped to packaging for flower or sent to a processor/extraction facility.
3. It is then sent to a manufacturer or company that will decide its fate. From there, the processed or semi-processed cannabis may be separated into various products.

*Note: 1st-party testing should be shipped with the biomass in order to "prove" you are delivering, shipping, and (the next link in the supply chain is) receiving a specific product, whether it be hemp or recreational cannabis.*

## Processing, extraction, and testing.

Processing and extraction facilities should receive the results of the 1st party testing prior to purchasing the biomass. From there, they would confirm that the product they receive has matching test results. The next step would be an initial crude extraction process, done by pressure, heat, solvents, or any combination thereof.

The product that results is typically a thick and dark brownish liquid. Its consistency comes from not yet being filtered, so it is still full of plant waxes, flavonoids, terpenes, chlorophyll, and other plant particles. Along with these, the raw, or acid form of the cannabinoids can be found. For hemp plants, this should bring the CBD (or CBDa, if no heat has been applied) concentration to roughly 35-55%.

The next potential step in the refining process for oils, vape cartridges, tinctures, or edibles is likely winterization. This can happen before or after decarboxylation. Depending on the goal of the brand or end user, the more concentrated the product is, the more steps are involved in the refinement process.

A very general breakdown of the cannabinoid content based on the way it is processed can be summarized as follows:

- Bud/Flower: 18%-22%

-smokable in bongs, pipes, joints, cones, blunts, herb vapes, and used to make cannabutter or infused in oils for edibles.

- Crude/Raw & Unfiltered extract: 40%-50%

Used to make waxes, dabs, and shatter, each has its own type of processing and filtration. They can be used for edibles, but they are not ideal.

- Post Decarboxylation & Winterization: 60%-70%
- Distillation: Distillate 80%-85%

Used for making oils, tinctures (full-spectrum or broad-spectrum), topicals, and liquid vape cartridges, it is easy to blend with oils or butter for edibles.

- After Remediation—Isolate 98%+

—(also known as pharmaceutical grade), used in formulation for anything that distillate can be used for but is in powder form. Any cannabinoid can be found in an "isolate" form, but CBD is the most common.

After processing, a second round of testing should be conducted by the refinery/extraction manufacturer. This round of testing should be a "full panel," meaning that it should be tested for cannabinoid content, terpene content (unless it went through remediation), molds and mycotoxins, bacteria, pesticides, and residual solvents. This round of testing is called 2nd party testing and will go to the party/company/manufacturer that will create the "end" product.

Once the end product is complete (for example, gummies or a massage oil), it gets tested a third time for final cannabinoid content. This indicates the amount of cannabinoids (such as CBD) that are in the final product. A final round of testing may conclude that there are 1500 mg of CBD in a one-ounce bottle of CBD oil or that there are 100 mg THC in a bag of sour hard candies, at 10 mg each. The third round of testing, at this point, should be conducted by an outside, independent, accredited laboratory in order to prevent any conflicts of interest. The results of this testing for safety, purity, and potency come in the form of a Certificate of Analysis (COA).

This last round of testing is called 3rd party Lab Testing. It is the "gold standard" when it comes to proving the quality and safety of a cannabis product. Some states require this for all products sold. Additional quality standards can come in the form of certification of processes and/or ingredients. Examples include Certified Organic, Kosher, cGMP, ISO 9001, and so on.

## Winterization (Sometimes Called Dewaxing)

This precise process involves dissolving the cannabis extract in a solvent (usually alcohol-based, like ethanol, hexane, or isopropanol), then chilling this mixture to a low temperature (ideally -4°F) in order to precipitate out impurities, such as lipids and waxes. The frozen mixture is then filtered, and the solvents are removed through evaporation and/or distillation. When done well, this leaves behind a cleaner, more concentrated liquid. It will be a thinner (and easier to work with) viscosity afterward. A couple of benefits to this include:

- Improved bioavailability is achieved by breaking down the plant material a little further, making it more absorbable by the body.
- Improved shelf life makes it less prone to oxidation and degradation.

When the winterization is ill-timed, improper temperatures, or too harsh solvents are used, it can reflect on the quality and safety of the final product. There are also some potential drawbacks of improper techniques that include:

- Loss of terpenes: high-boiling-point terpenes like myrcene and limonene may evaporate or degrade in the process.
- Residual solvents that can linger in the extract.
- THCa may also evaporate out in this process, reducing the THC potency once it has gone through decarboxylation.

Home processing operations don't typically take this step, as the equipment is expensive, it can be risky (utilizing highly flammable solvents), and it is overall more practical for large-scale production.

## Decarboxylation

*Decarb, or decarbing for short,* is the application of heat in order to "activate" or convert acidic forms of cannabinoids into "active" (sometimes referred to as *neutral* forms) to maximize the benefits. Decarbing can happen during various phases of processing, depending on the desired outcome. More recent research has shown that CBDa is, in fact, a more potent version of CBD. While THCa *won't* get you high, it still offers therapeutic benefits, as seen in the chart in Chapter 7.

The cannabinoid acid conversions include: THCa → Δ9THC, CBDa → CBD, CBGa → CBG, and CBCa → CBC. Ideal temperatures and times depend on the cannabinoid being converted, but here are some popular times and temperatures for the two major cannabinoids, CBD and THC:

CBDa → CBD: 130°C (266°F) for 20 min.

THCa → Δ9THC: 110°C (230°F) for 30–45 minutes.

This can "technically" happen during the distillation phase in commercial operations. Typically, higher quality products have been decarbed fully *prior* to distillation. Home growers and those who make cannabis edibles out of flower will typically do this by baking flower/bud in the oven. They do this after first breaking it down into small pieces, although there are many countertop machines out there that allow "home cooks" to make cannabutter or infused oils, with the decarb step built into the machine's processes. Decarbing naturally happens when a product is smoked or vaped.

## Distillation

Distillation is the process of further refining the extract—typically once it has already been decarbed and winterized. It is the same process that crude oil would go through to make gasoline, kerosene, and jet fuel. The purpose of this is to further concentrate the liquid, creating a thinner consistency, about the consistency of syrup, and a purer extract that is easier to formulate with and has the most "activated" cannabinoids. Some distillates can be made through *chromatography*, which will be explained more in depth in the next section, as it is the predominant way that isolates are produced.

*Fractional distillation* is most commonly used for all types of cannabis—a process that separates liquid components based on their boiling points. It allows specific cannabinoids to be either removed, targeted, or mitigated. *"Broad Spectrum* CBD oil" is the perfect example of this. It is a hemp-derived CBD oil that has had all the THC removed. (The benefits of broad spectrum CBD oil will be discussed in Ch. 19.)

It is also through this process that one might reintroduce any terpenes or cannabinoids that may have been lost along the way, through evaporation or temperature changes. The product of distillation and the liquid result of chromatography are referred to as a *"distillate."* Distillates can be sold or purchased as is—typically in very small amounts for personal use due to their concentration. More commonly, though, distillates are diluted in a carrier oil (e.g., MCT or hemp seed) for "oils" or "tinctures," or utilized as a base ingredient for bakers or formulators.

## Remediation

Remediation takes refinement to the next level. This is a process that breaks the oil down into singular compounds. This process creates a pure form of cannabinoids that are typically 98%-99.9% pure. The term *remediation* means removal. Essentially it means removing the compound- a cannabinoid in our case, from the solution (such as a distillate). The process of remediation is usually done through chromatography or crystallization.

Crystallization can form an isolate when a solvent is added to a concentrated solution, such as a distillate. The CBD, or other cannabinoids, then form crystals as the solvent, such as hexane or pentane, evaporates. It is a less expensive way to create bulk isolates than chromatography, but it cannot be used for THC, since it doesn't crystallize very easily.

Chromatography works by separating compounds based on their chemical properties, such as molecule size or polarity, rather than boiling points, as fractional distillation does. It comes in several forms, each with its own advantages. Here is a brief rundown:

- High-Performance Liquid Chromatography (HPLC) is very precise, uses solvents, and is acid-friendly.
- Flash chromatography (FC)—quick, bulk batches—uses polarity to separate.

- Supercritical Fluid Chromatography (sometimes referred to as *"Supercritical $CO_2$ Extraction") is a* solventless (cleaner) and the most eco-friendly method for bulk processing.
- Gas Chromatography (GC) is quick, but it uses heat, so it doesn't work for any acid forms.
- Thin Layer Chromatography (TLC) is ideal for lab testing and identification, but it is not suitable for high-level purification or for extracting the isolated compounds as a form of processing.

By breaking the product down into singular cannabinoids, it becomes much easier to study the effects on the body. This makes it easier to pinpoint specific dosages without having other cannabinoids, flavonoids, terpenes, or other natural components "interfere" with the desired effect. Because of this level of concentration and purity, it is sometimes marketed as "pharmaceutical grade." There is always an ongoing debate between "purity" vs. "The Entourage Effect," which we will dive into in the last part of this book. In my opinion, there are definite benefits to both, but you will have to decide for yourself which method resonates best with you.

# PART III

# BUILDING CANNABIS INTELLIGENCE

THE SECRET BODY SYSTEM THAT NO ONE EVER TALKS ABOUT, YET EVERYONE HAS.

## CHAPTER NINE

# WHAT IS THE ENDOCANNABINOID SYSTEM?

Believe it or not, all vertebrates have an endocannabinoid system (ECS). It is a body system just like the skeletal system or circulatory system. However, it does have some unique features that make it special. It is a SUPERCOMMUNICATOR. It is made up of endocannabinoids, enzymes, and receptors that allow the body's other systems to communicate with each other through channels. It is often lumped in with the nervous system due to its ability to send messages throughout the body, using the nervous system as one of its many conduits for communication. It ebbs and flows with our body's natural cycles and is interwoven into the fabric of our being.

Its role in our body is to maintain homeostasis.

Balance.

Wellness.

Yep. It's a pretty big deal.

Have you ever had an injury? If so, your ECS was affected.

Do you have any diseases, disorders, or imbalances in your body? If so, your ECS is involved.

Have you ever experienced stress? Yep. Your ECS is leading the way to help cope with that too. (If you said NO to this one, I wouldn't believe you!) Your ECS is a regulator for all aspects of your health, regardless of cannabis usage. We were all designed to have a functioning endocannabinoid system from day one. It is an integral part of our immune function, digestion, endocrine system, nervous system, and the development of all the body's systems in one way or another. In utero, the mother and baby exchange fluid through the umbilical cord, including endocannabinoids. Research has also shown the ECS to suppress tumors in a targeted fashion for many types of cancer.

## Parts of the ECS

The ECS is made up of three parts.

1. **Endocannabinoids** are the cannabinoids naturally produced by our bodies. (Endo = internally produced.) So far, they have identified two endocannabinoids—both of which promote sleep and modulate anxiety.

*Anandamide (AEA), discovered* in 1992, is a fatty-acid neurotransmitter nicknamed the "Bliss Molecule." It creates the experience of "reward," regulating behavior and is also tied to the feeling of motivation, responsible for sensations such as the "runner's high." It bonds to the CB1 receptors, which trigger the chemical signals that modify behavior.

*2-Arachidonoylglycerol (2-AG)*- regulates the circulatory system directly and/or indirectly through metabolites when broken down. These affect the blood vessels and/or heart. They bond primarily to CB2 receptors and, to a lesser extent, to CB1 receptors. 2-AG may also act as a defense mechanism for the brain, with neuroprotective qualities that increase brain resilience in response to infection or injury.

2. **Cannabinoid Receptors**- specialized receptors that control physiological processes, including appetite, pain, mood, memory, nausea, and inflammation, regardless of cannabis use.

Both endocannabinoids, which are made by the body, and phytocannabinoids, which are derived from the plant, connect to these receptors in our bodies to produce a specific, desired effect on a bodily system.

These receptors are found in men, women, and animals. They are present in every body system and work together for the "common good." Endocannabinoid receptors utilize cannabinoids, proteins, and enzymes to send signals that bring the body into healthy balance or homeostasis.

In order of abundance, these are the known receptors engaged by cannabinoids:

*CB1 Receptors* connect to our central nervous system. They have an effect on and are also found in the following:

The brain and central nervous system (which includes the spinal cord and nerves)

The gastrointestinal tract (which includes the stomach and intestines)

→ Vascular system (which includes blood and the lymphatic vessels)

→ Muscles (including smooth muscles found around the organs)

→ Reproductive system (in both males and females, but more extensively in females)

*CB2 Receptors* run alongside the peripheral nervous system and are found in the:

→ Skin

→ Immune Cells

→ Bones

→ Spleen

→ Glial Cells

*Transient receptor potential (TRP) channels* are located on the cell surface, allowing cells to receive signals of environmental and sensory changes. TRP channels are located throughout the following:

- Nervous system (multiple processes including nerve cell growth and death, as well as synaptic transmissions)
- Skin (specifically, the microbiome)

- Digestive system (which monitors chemicals and toxins in food, digestive enzymes, and the gut microbiome)

*The peroxisome proliferator-activated receptor (PPAR)* has the main role of regulating metabolic function and energy levels, as well as keeping both balanced.

BOTH CB1 and CB2 Receptors are also found in the:

→ Lungs

→ Liver

→ Gallbladder

→ Pancreas

→ Bone marrow

→ Brain stem

In the case of TRP and PPAR, the connection and impact on receptors can occur when cannabinoids are assisted by fatty acid-binding proteins.

Example: If someone has oily skin, CBD usage can signal the body to reduce sebum production without completely shutting it off in order to bring the body into a healthy balance.

3. **Enzymes** are hugely responsible for the biosynthesis and metabolism of endocannabinoids.

There are two types that break down endocannabinoids once they are "spent":

- FAAH, short for fatty acid amide hydrolase, breaks down AEA. This means that after AEA is "used" by the CB1 receptors, it essentially deactivates.
- MAGL breaks down 2-AG into glycerol and fatty acid in the presynaptic terminal.

There are three enzymes responsible for synthesizing the endocannabinoids, and they are listed as follows:

1. NAPE synthesizes AEA, predominantly in the kidneys, which contributes to electrolyte and fluid homeostasis. However, the system responsible for this action still needs further research.
2. DAGL-α produces 2-AG in neurons, which directs nerve fiber growth within the brain and regulates learning and memory processes.
3. DAGL-β produces 2-AG in innate immune cells to control inflammatory lipid and protein signaling.

## How It Works

When the discovery of the ECS was publicized, beginning in the 1990s and continuing through about 2018, we were taught that cannabinoids would bind to receptors in a "lock and key" type system. This is now found to be only partially true.

Newer research shows more accuracy. Only cannabinoids that directly bind to the receptors act more like the "lock and key" mechanism. Both THC from cannabis and anandamide (AEA) do this with CB1 receptors.

CBD does not react in this way with CB1 and CB2 receptors, however. It does act *indirectly* on cannabinoid receptors. Instead of the "lock and key" or on/off type of interaction, it works more like a "flow valve." Instead of CBD telling these parts to either "work" or "shut down" (such as in the lock and key theory), the receptors instead act as a flow mediator, like a water valve. This "valve" controls the input and output of chemical and electrical signals that regulate the body's systems and bring them into balance.

According to the lists of locations of cannabinoid receptors, you will notice that all the body systems are tied to the ECS. The organs that are not *directly* tied to the endocannabinoid system are connected to it *indirectly* through the HPA axis.

For those who remember how the HPA axis works, this may sound familiar. The following is a quick rundown:

In the HPA axis, the 'H' stands for hypothalamus, the 'P' stands for pituitary, and the 'A' stands for adrenal. All three parts rely on each other in a feedback loop to constantly boost or suppress the hormones and nerve signals that course through your body. Now, I'm not just talking about reproductive hormones, although they are in charge of that too; I am talking about cortisol (the stress hormone) levels, blood sugar (energy) levels, and so much more!

The hypothalamus acts as a mediator for both chemical and electrical signals. It is a small region of the brain that "gives orders" for glands (such as the pituitary gland and the adrenals) to release hormones and regulate neurotransmitter responses. This type of regulation is crucial for healthy brain functions and bodily processes. It has six primary duties in the body, and they are BIG roles.

1. Endocrine control regulates growth, metabolism, and reproduction.
2. Autonomic Nervous System Control—which controls involuntary functions such as heart rate, breathing, blood pressure, and digestion—is also responsible for the "fight or flight" response.
3. Homeostasis maintains body temperature, fluid levels, and electrolyte balance.
4. Behavior and emotion regulate mood, sleep cycles, and appetite.
5. Growth and development are active, especially during puberty.
6. The stress response releases cortisol, adrenaline, and other stress-related hormones.

"Wait, what?! Don't many of those duties overlap with the endocannabinoid system?" you may ask. Yep. Even homeostasis and physiological processes like appetite and mood do.

Often known as the "master control center," the hypothalamus is a MAJOR producer of endocannabinoids.

It is also home to MANY CB1 receptors, as they are a part of the brain. Our friend, the hypothalamus, is even responsible for non-hormone-based tasks, such as pain perception, memory, and learning. These, in turn, are affected by the cannabinoids, both endo- and phyto-. By having appropriate levels of cannabinoids in our body's endocannabinoid system, these regulatory tasks can remain "in balance" with each other. When these processes, chemicals, or feedback loops are not functioning properly, diseases and disorders arise. These symptoms, of varying types, start appearing to signal that something is wrong.

That being said, men and women were each designed with their own unique anatomy and body chemistry. This explains why our bodies react differently to various stimuli and the differing needs on a very basic level. Men and women need different amounts of optimal sleep, activity, and nutrients (including protein and minerals), as well as recovery time. The next chapter will cover some of the key differences in the endocannabinoid system between the genders.

## CHAPTER TEN

# BIOLOGICAL DIFFERENCES IN THE ECS: MEN VS. WOMEN

On a biological level, men and women have some differences in their endocannabinoid systems and how they function. Some of the key differences lie in the way women's bodies are specifically designed to carry out the function of childbirth and in the way each sex reacts to stressors.

Our hormones, both reproductive and those involved in energy levels, stress response, metabolism, and development, all impact the way our bodies interact with cannabinoids. There are differences in how hormones interact with endocannabinoids, body composition, and also in the location and number of cannabinoid receptors that are unique to each sex.

## Hormonal Influence

The female ECS is directly influenced by fluctuating levels of estrogen and progesterone throughout the menstrual cycle. Estrogen, in particular, has been shown to increase the levels of endocannabinoids like anandamide. THC doesn't interact with estrogen receptors, nor do any other cannabinoids, with the exception of a very high concentration of

CBD in a study called "Marijuana: Interaction with the Estrogen Receptor."

In contrast, the male ECS is less affected by hormone fluctuations since testosterone levels tend to be more stable. Not only that, but the amount of phytoestrogens *(or plant-derived estrogens)* produced by the cannabis plant is very low—much lower than that of flax seeds, soy, beer, and coffee.

Keep in mind that when cannabis is in a concentrated, whole plant/full spectrum, or resinous form, the phytoestrogens become more potent. Heavy use of concentrated forms of cannabis ***can*** impact the phytoestrogen levels for both sexes.

## Cannabinoid Receptor Density

Studies suggest that females may have a higher density of cannabinoid receptors (CB1 and CB2) in certain regions of the brain, leading to a more pronounced effect when cannabinoids are consumed. This could explain why women may experience stronger effects of cannabinoids in areas like pain relief or mood regulation. In addition to that, there are more endocannabinoid receptors found in the female reproductive system than in the male system.

## Stress Response

There is evidence suggesting that the ECS responds differently to stress in men and women. Females may have a more sensitive ECS when it comes to managing stress, anxiety, and mood regulation due to the interactions between estrogen and endocannabinoid signaling. This can influence how women experience anxiety and depression, particularly during hormonal shifts, such as menstruation or menopause.

### Sensitivity to Cannabinoids

Women may be more sensitive to the pain-relieving and psychoactive effects of cannabinoids, like THC, due to hormonal interactions. On the other hand, men tend to show different responses related to motor control and reward pathways, which could be influenced by testosterone.

### Effect of Cannabinoid Use

Research has indicated that chronic cannabis use can have different impacts on males and females, especially regarding cognition and addiction potential in the psychoactive forms (especially THC). Some studies suggest that males may develop tolerance faster due to having fewer endocannabinoid receptors and experience different behavioral and cognitive changes compared to females.

Females may be more susceptible than males to the anxiogenic (anxiety-producing) effects of THC. It is also worth noting that women tend to self-medicate with cannabis for mood disorders such as anxiety and depression more frequently than men.

### BMI—Body Mass Index

Plant cannabinoids (phytocannabinoids) are fat-soluble. On average, women have higher body fat content than men in order to support reproduction. Because of this, women tend to store cannabinoids, such as CBD, for longer in their body's adipose (fatty) tissues. This allows women to supplement with cannabinoids less often or at lower doses once their ECS is regulated. (We will discuss this more in Part 4: "The Ultimate Dosing Guide.")

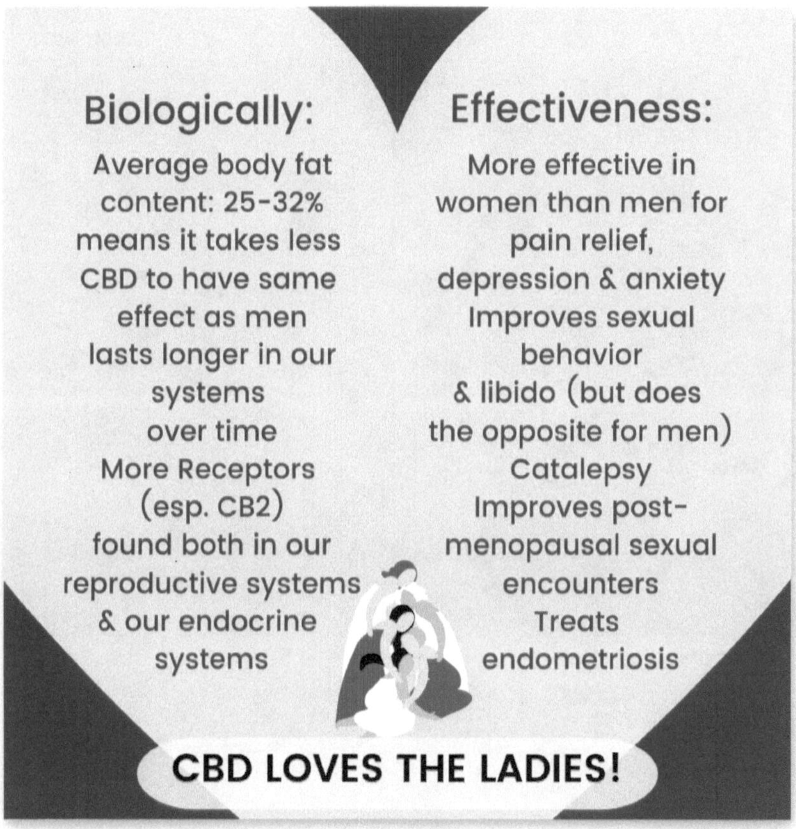


While the ECS functions similarly in both sexes, hormonal fluctuations and receptor distribution make its effects gender-specific in many ways. Knowing this, we can be better informed on how to modify our cannabinoid usage. This affects dosing, tolerance, the duration of time that cannabinoids circulate throughout the body, the potential for addiction, and even the occurrence of dysfunction in the ECS. Therefore, by taking into account these biological differences, we are better able to support a healthy ECS, build resilience, and age more gracefully.

# CHAPTER ELEVEN

# WHAT HAPPENS IF THE ECS ISN'T WORKING PROPERLY?

Chances are, the first signs that your endocannabinoid system is dysfunctioning will be subtle. Maybe you are catching every cold that goes around the office and just assume it's because it's "flu season." Or possibly you're struggling to sleep well and blame it on a stressful week. Or maybe you're waking up achy and just chalking it up to "getting older." While those things are valid on their own, the collaborative effort between the ECS and the body (wellness) can be interrupted by injury, toxins, trauma, or unmanaged stress. This isolates the body from regaining homeostasis. These imbalances could eventually lead to illness or disease.

Anyone can have a deficiency in endocannabinoids—

Compounds naturally produced in the body help regulate various physiological functions, including mood, pain, appetite, and sleep. This deficiency could be linked to several chronic conditions, and all of these conditions can be tied to HPA Axis Dysregulation. This refers to an imbalance in the activity of the hypothalamic-pituitary-adrenal

(HPA) axis, the body's primary stress response system, which we learned about at the end of Chapter 9.

The endocannabinoid system plays a crucial role in regulating this axis, acting as a natural "brake" to help dampen excessive stress responses. Essentially, a dysregulated HPA axis can be partially corrected by a properly functioning endocannabinoid system. An effectively functioning ECS can help mitigate the effects of chronic stress by modulating the release of stress hormones like cortisol. Researchers are now seeing many links between these deficiencies and conditions with unknown causes.

Endocannabinoid system challenges can present early on as common symptoms of stress, exhaustion, and/or generalized anxiety. When this has been left untreated, it frequently leads to:

- Chronic inflammatory conditions
- An underactive or overactive immune system.
- Insomnia
- Gut issues
- Pain

It is possible, even probable, that you may experience some or all of those symptoms either independently or together, but not necessarily all the time.

***There are seven major risk factors that can (and do) affect ECS functioning and cannabinoid deficiency.***

Some of these factors overlap (e.g., toxin exposure can cause inflammation). Others are a result of environmental elements, lifestyle choices, and even factors beyond one's control.

1. **Genetics:** Some people may naturally produce fewer endocannabinoids or have fewer cannabinoid receptors due to their genetic makeup.

2. **Chronic Stress**: Long-term stress can deplete the body's endocannabinoid levels, reducing the effectiveness of the endocannabinoid system (ECS).

3. **Poor Diet**: A diet low in essential fatty acids, which are precursors to endocannabinoids, may result in a lower production of these compounds.

4. **Lack of Physical Activity**: Exercise can boost endocannabinoid levels, so a sedentary lifestyle might contribute to a deficiency.

5. **Toxin Exposure**: Environmental toxins, such as heavy metals or pollutants, may disrupt the balance of the ECS.

6. **Chronic Inflammation**: Inflammatory conditions can interfere with the functioning of the ECS, potentially leading to imbalances.

7. **Aging**: As people age, their endocannabinoid system may become less efficient, leading to lower levels of endocannabinoids.

Any one of these things can cause problems with your appetite, mood, pain levels, or quality of sleep, but the more risk factors you have, the worse your condition may become. It may even lead to a chronic condition referred to as "clinical endocannabinoid deficiency."

## Endocannabinoid System Dysfunction

CECD (Clinical Endocannabinoid Deficiency) is a research-supported theory that arose in 2016. It suggests that over time, ECS dysfunction could be the cause of conditions such as fibromyalgia, migraines, IBS, and a few other conditions, including several neurological disorders that have no clear underlying cause. These conditions also tend to be resistant to treatment and sometimes occur alongside one another. Major signs of ECS deficiency are high levels of oxidative stress, a lack of or poor sleep, and anxiety.

There are 4 potential ways that the ECS can become inhibited, causing dysfunction in the body to the point of CECD:

***1. Not enough CB receptors.***

Without enough "connectors," the signals can't get to their designated areas. There is a plethora of reasons for a lack of endocannabinoid receptors in the body.

Example: Let's say there are not enough endocannabinoid receptors in the stomach. The stomach sends signals to the brain to either be hungry or full (potentially "satisfied").

These signals are not being sent properly, so the person may not "feel full", and unintentionally overeat. Overeating can then lead to several serious issues, including obesity, type 2 diabetes, heart disease, and eventually heart failure. If addressed early on, these more serious complications can be prevented.

***2. Too many metabolic enzymes.***

An excess of these enzymes could potentially break down the endocannabinoids or cannabinoids before they reach the receptors and are fully utilized by the body. Think of it like running a marathon but drinking all of your water during the warm-up and still needing more halfway through the race.

***3. Synthesizing insufficient AEA and 2-AG.***

This can happen when the body is creating deformed, weak, or not enough endocannabinoids. In Chapter 10, we learned about the endocannabinoids that help control systems in our body that regulate our feelings of "reward" as well as motivation.

Of these particular cannabinoids, AEA is concentrated in the CB1 receptors in the brain. The other well-known endocannabinoid, 2-AG, is important for our circulatory system, helping to regulate our heart and blood flow. These are found mostly in the CB2 receptors, with only a few affecting the CB1 receptors.

These endocannabinoids are also responsible for a balanced immune response, as well as proper neuron function, which is essential for learning and memory processes in the brain.

E*xample: What happens when you are deficient in AEA? It can cause stress-induced anxiety and even lead to depression.*

***4. Incomplete connections***

The receptor site may not make a solid connection between endocannabinoids and CB receptors due to poor signaling or improper attachment. They could be deformed receptors, oddly shaped endocannabinoids, or the signal may not have reached the intended source. It is also common for toxins, drugs, and even medications—which we will discuss more in Part 4—to block the connections, signaling pathways, and/or the synthesis of endocannabinoids. Example: The cytochrome P450 (CYP) enzyme family is responsible for metabolizing a multitude of medications, as well as both endo- and phyto-cannabinoids. There are MANY common medications that share the same pathways for metabolism. (See list in Appendix I.)

The exact causes of CECD are not fully understood, but long-term or extreme cases of the seven major risk factors listed earlier can lead to one or more of the 4 ways that the endo-cannabinoid system can become injured or dysfunctional.

You can have CECD and still have other health conditions as well. In fact, this is extremely common. Testing the ECS directly isn't yet widely known or standardized in medical practice. However, research into CECD is ongoing, and there are a few ways to potentially assess endocannabinoid system function, including:

**Blood Tests -** Researchers can measure levels of endocannabinoids (like anandamide or 2-AG) and their metabolites in the blood. These specialized tests are mostly used in research settings rather than clinical settings.

**Symptom Tracking** – Since CECD is believed to be connected to conditions like chronic pain, migraines, or gastrointestinal disorders, tracking symptoms and correlating them with possible ECS dysfunction may provide insight.

**Genetic Testing-** Some companies offer genetic testing to examine variations in genes related to the ECS. These variations might affect how your body produces and uses endocannabinoids.

**Research Studies -** Participating in research studies focused on the ECS could offer a more direct way of assessing your endocannabinoid system and determining if CECD might be a factor in your health.

If you're interested in exploring the possibility of CECD or understanding more about your endocannabinoid system, it might be helpful to consult with a healthcare provider who is experienced in cannabinoid medicine. They can offer insights into how ECS dysfunction could be influencing your health and what steps you might take.

If you are noticing that you are experiencing unexplained chronic inflammatory conditions, immune system challenges, insomnia, gut issues, and/or pain, then consider what you can do to start supporting your ECS. You'll learn how, in the next few chapters, either with or without cannabinoid supplementation.

# CHAPTER TWELVE

## HOW DO I SUPPORT MY ECS?

Nobody likes to hear it, but as with most worthwhile endeavors, supporting your endocannabinoid system takes work. Not everyone has the same privileges when it comes to where they live, what products they use, and the circumstances of their daily life. We ALL struggle in some aspect of our lives, in SOME way. None of us are immune to stress. Everyone has some form of trauma, challenge, disability, conflict, disease, hardship, and/or setback they must overcome. We are only human.

~BUT~

We are intricately and intentionally designed to survive, even THRIVE, despite these stressors in our lives. Although diet and exercise play an important role in the wellness of your endocannabinoid system, a more holistic, multifaceted approach will create a sustainable and effective way to heal and improve ECS function.

***There is no magic pill.***

While Western medicine has had amazing advances in trauma care, surgeries, and technology, it is most frequently utilized to "manage symptoms" as opposed to finding a root cause and healing the issues. Medications, both pharmaceutical and over-the-counter, can be great at providing short-term relief but are often not intended for long-term use.

Both long- and short-term medications can, and often do, impact your body in unintended ways. Liver damage, kidney failure, stomach ulcers, and digestive issues are all very common side effects of using medications frequently. Ironically, more often than not, it usually is not providing a "cure" for the ailment.

Addiction, paralysis, and even death are also commonly listed as potential issues from pharmaceutical intervention, yet Western culture has deemed these as an "acceptable risk" for managing health issues. In fact, the U.S. has a long track record of "hidden agendas" when it comes to the pharmaceutical, petrochemical, and insurance industries, but that is for a different book.

Even "safe" and life-saving medications, such as antibiotics, can have a negative impact on one's health by killing beneficial gut bacteria. Short-term effects can be noticed as nausea and/or poor digestion (constipation, bloating), whereas long-term or frequent usage can result in antibiotic resistance, psychiatric diseases, cardiovascular disease, and even cancer, especially colon cancer.

As far as I know, there is no current *medication* aimed specifically at supporting the endocannabinoid system. There are SEVERAL medications out there that offer (synthetic) cannabinoids as a treatment for specific conditions: Marinol, Syndros, Sativex, and Cesamet. There is only one that is derived from natural sources—Epidiolex, which is made from CBD isolate and is only prescribed for Lennox-Gastaut syndrome, Dravet syndrome, or tuberous sclerosis (all are severe forms of epilepsy). Pharmaceutical regulations don't allow "off-label" prescriptions.

Thankfully, due to the 2018 Farm Bill and the federal legalization of hemp, cannabinoids that are safe and accessible for supplementation are now plentiful. Many states, since 2012, have also joined in on the legal cannabis trend by fully legalizing recreational cannabis on a state-by-state basis. The challenge remains, though, in the education surrounding the legal cannabinoids available, especially in the CBD and THC markets.

Although there are still plenty of boomers out there with sage advice on their experience with ganja from their hippie era, today's recreational cannabis is not your mama's weed. It is bred and hybridized to be WAY more potent, and there are many new methods of consumption, as well as unique processing methods, that just weren't even dreamt up yet in their day. There are definitely still some traditionalists out there who are growing a version of their favorite strains, like "Acapulco Gold" or "Afghani," which were popular when they were younger. There is still plenty of opportunity to consume cannabis in the classic ways—smoking a joint, pipe, or blunt, hitting a bong; or devouring some hash brownies. However, modern processing methods offer additional options to indulge in cannabinoid consumption. You can buy THC sodas, CBN vape pens, Delta-8 gummies, or even CBD toothpaste! The options are practically endless. The rest of this book is aimed at guiding you through the process of regaining control of your health by supporting your ECS in a way that is right for YOU.

Luckily, there are ways you can, and should, support and heal your endocannabinoid system *without* having to add cannabinoids to your routine. However, in many cases, supplementation can help jumpstart the process to a healthier, happier, and more resilient state of being. Here is a story of someone who did just that.

## The Story of Sara

This story is an example of somebody (we'll call her Sara) who wanted to use the CBD-based medication Epidiolex for anxiety. Sara knew how beneficial CBD could be for this; however, a doctor couldn't prescribe her that medication for it.

Not prescribing a medication for anxiety (even CBD) is a blessing in disguise, though! Anxiety is typically a symptom of one or more underlying causes. The root issues can be addressed while still treating the symptom of anxiety strictly by making lifestyle shifts that can contribute to long-term health and stress management. These root issues may include a poor diet, not enough sunlight, repressed emotions, improper stress management, and/or a lack of exercise. Sara can change and ideally optimize these things to boost the body's natural endocannabinoids. As an added bonus, if she turns these actions into lifelong habits, she will benefit from a stronger immune system and overall longevity.

More often than not, aspects of anxiety can also stem from past or current trauma. According to Dr. Francine Shapiro, who developed the treatment "Eye Movement Desensitization and Reprocessing" (EMDR), she describes trauma in two ways:

1. The "Big T" trauma, or severe distress, is caused by major life events, such as losing a home in a natural disaster, experiencing a personal assault, or the loss of a child.
2. A "small t" trauma can refer to a less severe but still impactful trauma, such as consistent criticism, a breakup, the death of a pet, or financial hardship.

No matter what form of trauma has been experienced, counseling can be an integral part of healing to fully address long-term or chronic anxiety.

CBD supplementation may still be necessary until Sara gets into a healthy routine of managing her anxiety naturally, but it can still happen, luckily, thanks to the hemp laws. As a bonus, Sara will now gain a LOT more benefits from these natural "treatments" than she would have from the standard, commonly prescribed medications for anxiety. She also won't have the common side effects of:

- Drowsiness
- Upset stomach
- Weight gain
- Dry mouth
- Sexual problems
- Headaches
- Blurred vision
- Mood changes
- Dizziness
- Confusion

She also won't be risking potential addiction to the frequently prescribed SSRIs. Yet, by utilizing the "alternative treatments," she will likely experience the side effects of a stronger immune system, improved mood, healthier digestion, better sleep, reduced inflammation, and a more resilient endocannabinoid system! Don't get me wrong; cannabis products can have side effects as well, and we will discuss those. However, it has been recognized worldwide as a safe and effective treatment for a multitude of issues. Typically, the "side effects" can be avoided with the right type of product and dosage for you and your condition.

Many biohackers, naturopaths, functional medicine providers, Eastern medicine doctors, indigenous medicine men (and women), and integrative medicine practitioners would agree that a multifaceted wellness plan should include mind, body, and spirit. This will improve your chances of reversing most diseases and disorders. There are a multitude of books, podcasts, and YouTube videos on this type of approach, and I will include several examples in the *Resources* section at the back of this book.

It is the mindfulness of how we choose to treat our bodies, and the way we manage our emotions, work through trauma, participate in relationships, along with the habits we practice daily, that will either lead to wellness or disorder. This list of lifestyle factors is not all-inclusive, but it does outline a good starting point. This list can give you a place to begin addressing areas of your life that can be examined in order to support a strong, healthy, and highly functioning endocannabinoid system.

- Environment
- Lifestyle
- Mental Health Management
- Nutrition

Each of these topics deserves its own book on ways the strategy can optimize wellness. Every shift can impact your well-being either positively or negatively. There is ample, in-depth research regarding the implementation of the strategies that I'll highlight in the next chapter.

Each of these areas should be addressed before adding cannabis to your life. Why before? With these new habits in place, the body will be primed to function at a much higher level! Once in practice, the need for supplementation with cannabis and/or other vitamins, minerals, and essential nutrients will likely become drastically reduced and/or changed to an "as needed" scenario, depending on the level of health challenges you are currently facing.

You have already taken the first step in this leg of the journey by reading this book, learning about the function of the ECS, and gaining an awareness of some of the potential that cannabis holds. By putting effort into a holistic approach, not solely relying on supplements and/or medications to give your body the healing support it needs, you will discover even further hidden benefits.

*A more meaningful sense of purpose.*
*Inner peace and joy.*
*Success.*
*Fulfillment.*

# CHAPTER THIRTEEN

# SETTING THE STAGE FOR A STRONGER ECS

How do you support a body system you didn't even know you had? Believe it or not, it is more straightforward than you would think, summed up in one 6- letter word: *stress.*

As you learned in previous chapters, our mind and our body are separate but highly intertwined parts of the same system. The parts work together, in checks and balances, through feedback loops, electrical signals, chemical signals, and reactions; the communication that happens between all the body's systems is supported by the endocannabinoid system. This system is highly influenced by everything we are exposed to; unmanaged stress is a quick way for dysfunction to rear its ugly head.

Now, before you start thinking that "stress" should be a four-letter word, hear me out. Stress is a natural, useful, unavoidable, and essential part of life. It builds resilience, inspires innovation, demands action, motivates, and spurs creativity. This positive form of stress is called *"eustress."*

Eustress comes in the form of a competitive athlete pushing their body to the limit during training. It is the high school valedictorian prepping for her speech. It is the executive negotiating with an investor or a grandparent babysitting their toddler grandchild. Eustress can be joyful, rewarding, beneficial, and even manageable.

Stress comes in MANY forms and as you know, not all stress is beneficial to our lives. Negative stress, unresolved stress, and unnecessary stress and worse. We know this as *distress*. Things we think of as distress can include a car accident, bankruptcy, a fight with your spouse, a sick pet, someone insulting you, heavy traffic, deadlines, or losing your cell phone. Things we may not think of as stress include the media, a messy workspace, our negative self-talk, artificial fragrances, our frenemies, and even excessive exercise.

We all experience both eustress and distress. How stress affects our lives and endocannabinoid system is dependent on how long it lasts, the amount of time it takes to resolve, and its intensity.

Short-term stress happens quickly and typically ends quickly. Short-term stress may be as simple as running late for work or seeing a spider crawling toward your plate at dinner. Some stress is a result of our own choices, such as over-booking our schedules or going to a job interview. Other times, it is out of our control, such as getting cut off while driving.

Short-term, or *acute stress*, can happen frequently, taking a long-term toll on our system. This is referred to as *"episodic acute stress."* It can happen to anyone and typically takes the form of leading a chaotic lifestyle. The blessing is that this can be reversed. *Chronic stress*, of either type, persists over an extended period of time—weeks, months, or possibly even years. This type of stress can lead to major health issues—ones that are potentially irreversible. Yes, even eustress can lead to burnout, neglecting self-care, and an unhealthy amount of risk-taking.

We were designed to respond to stress, adapt, and/or heal and move on. We need to strike a healthy balance and manage ALL types of stress. A good first step in managing stress is recognizing where it comes from and being aware of the various forms of it that can affect our well-being.

Stress comes at us from all different angles and sources. It is steeped in our surroundings, the way we live, our experiences, memories, food, beliefs, relationships, and careers. I've categorized them into three basic categories: physical, lifestyle, and mental health.

I've broken them down in a basic way to give a brief overview of how various factors can influence stress and, therefore, your endocannabinoid system. All the categories have crossovers. All categories are not proportionate to each individual. There will be topics that are completely irrelevant for some. Some are born into more stressful lives than others. No one can avoid stress, but everyone can make the most of the things they have control over. First - awareness, second - mindful shifts, third - building new habits, until one has made enough changes to achieve balance, well-being, joy and purpose.

## #1 Physical and #2 Lifestyle

*Physical* refers to not only the physical demands on the body and of the body but also to what the physical body is exposed to from the environment.

*Lifestyle* encompasses everything about the way one lives, including how you treat your physical body (which is why I included it in this physical section). It also includes your daily habits, attitude, outlook, social influences, and financial commitments. Your lifestyle affects your mental health, and vice versa—they are all interconnected.

Environment: What we hear, see, smell, taste, and touch. What is more prevalent in your life—air pollution or fresh ocean air? Birds chirping or emergency sirens? Sunshine or fluorescent lighting?

Safety: A sense of safety can impact your nervous system and stress levels in a big way. Safety from physical harm and emotional trauma, through bullying and/or verbal abuse, is an aspect of stress that bleeds into all the categories affecting relationships, physical health, and mental health.

Needs: The quality of water, foods, and all consumables, including vitamins, supplements, medications, smoking, and/or vaping, must be taken into consideration when it comes to the impact of stress on the body. Do you know whether the foods you are eating are relieving stress, like almonds, or contributing to oxidative stress, like Oreos? (We'll go over nutrition in the next chapter.) Are you moving your body? If so, how? Do you sit for the majority of the day? Do you vary your movement? Do you lift heavy things with proper body mechanics?

Ideally, one would replace negative physical stressors with positive ones, but life isn't always transactional like that. Some things will take time to change, while other things can be incorporated today! Here is a list of ideas to get you started:

- Watching the sunrise and sunset or watching flames in a safe environment (i.e., fireplace, bonfire, and/or candlelight).
- Positive consensual touch (i.e., hugs, hand-holding, high fives, massage, back scratching, tickling, snuggling, kissing, and/or sex)
- Hydrotherapy (i.e., Epsom salt baths, bubble baths, steam rooms, cold plunges, float tanks—sensory deprivation, hot tubbing, and/or getting in the ocean)
- "Touching grass" (i.e., grounding/earthing, forest bathing, gardening, caring for houseplants, smelling/looking at flowers, exploring botanical gardens, spending time at a park, camping, and/or beach time)
- Music that makes you happy (i.e., humming, singing, wind chimes, nature sounds including fountains, waterfalls, ocean waves, and/or birds chirping). Sound healing, such as theta wave frequency healing (known as Solfeggio frequencies),

involves specific sound frequencies used to promote healing and well-being—444 Hz is associated with emotional healing and balance, 396 is tied to liberating guilt, fear, and trauma, and 528 is known as the love frequency. Other types of traditional sound therapies are Tibetan sound bowls and crystal singing bowls.

- Movement is medicine—being mindful of your body's limitations while still engaging your muscles and giving your heart a workout does triple duty: it manages stress, releases endorphins, and releases toxins through sweat! It is an extremely underutilized tool, and it doesn't have to cost anything. Walking, dancing, exercising, martial arts, hula hooping, bike riding, playing tag, swimming, jumping rope, swinging on a swing set, hiking, and/or climbing a tree (be careful)! Other activities include playing tug of war or fetch with your pet (with bonus exercise for your pooch)!

## #3: Mental (and Spiritual) Health

There are a lot of topics and areas of focus that can be included under the heading of mental health: psychological, emotional, theological, relational, and/or spiritual.

Within these, healthy ways to seek a stronger mental capacity can include an assortment of avenues that, again, work together. Emotional regulation, trauma support, mindfulness, building self-worth, mental stimulation (both through learning and creativity), and adopting healthy coping mechanisms are all worthy of your attention.

Mental health is not just a hot topic but a potentially *life-saving* pursuit. For some, this means seeking the meaning of life—purpose, knowing their creator, or having no regrets. For others, it means mending fences in relationships, reassessing their spiritual beliefs, and checking things off the bucket list. Addressing all the things that have been put off for "later" now becomes important when a life-changing diagnosis occurs.

Two big areas come to mind when it comes to finding a sense of mental peace and clarity: addressing unresolved issues and managing stress well.

Addressing unresolved issues through counseling, prioritizing who and what is important in your life, including exploring your faith, identifying toxic relationships, and eliminating or reducing the time spent with those people can all be a great way to offload emotional, social, and mental health stressors. Our will to live and move forward directly affects our body's ability to heal. *Research suggests a potential link between suppressed anger and the development or progression of certain cancers (breast, prostate, lung, and colorectal). Be sure to examine:*

- Relationship with your higher power. What do you believe? Are you living in alignment with that? Do you need to go deeper?
- Your relationships with others—learning and

practicing effective communication, setting healthy boundaries, practicing giving grace, making amends, and providing and asking for forgiveness.
- The relationship you have with yourself by: eliminating negative self-talk, practicing gratitude, letting go of resentment, working through past trauma, and examining your own guilt and shame.

Stress management When you manage your stress better, you allow yourself to experience more joy. Stress management doesn't have to be expensive or complicated. Feel free to think outside the box. Sure, you can binge a Netflix series, but let's get creative.

- Learn what helps you relax: massage, meditation, walks, listening to music, good conversation with friends, playing in the dirt, breathwork, a nap, playing with or snuggling your pet, exercising, laying out in the sunshine, laughing, dancing, singing, intimate time with your partner, a phone call or FaceTime with a loved one, cooking or baking, silly animal videos, daydreaming—the list is endless and individualized.
- Have fun. Play. It may be something that is a bit taxing on your body but truly helps release endorphins and serotonin, relaxing your mind or providing emotional release. Some examples of this include hitting a punching bag, running, practicing martial arts, hitting golf balls, riding bikes, bowling,

hiking, playing a game of tag, jumping on a trampoline, playing video games, going to a shooting range, and playing games like "Chess," "Cornhole," or "Cards Against Humanity."
- Mental play—journaling, learning a new language, creativity in art, coloring, knitting/crocheting, playing with clay or playdough, taking a class for fun, shooting photography, putting together puzzles, or trying out an escape room—can all be done as solitary activities or with others.

These steps to strengthen your endocannabinoid system, along with the advice in the next chapter about nutrition, could lead to a healthy lifestyle, but also to a more fulfilled and joyful sense of being. When you are less stressed, healthier, and have stronger relationships, good things tend to happen. You have more capacity to grow as a person, reach your goals, and gain opportunities for greater personal and financial success.

# CHAPTER FOURTEEN

# NUTRITION, STRESS, AND THE GUT-BRAIN CONNECTION

The final piece of advice on balancing the endocannabinoid system lies in nutrition, which includes drinks, herbs, and supplements. Not only is food a basic daily need, but it is also woven into every culture as a social activity. It can be a part of our religious and/or personal belief systems and is a powerful tool to either heal or harm the body.

We overindulge during celebrations. We eat our feelings. We self-soothe with sweets and alcohol. We diet. We fast. We supplement, restrict, and we often don't even know what we are putting into our bodies.

There is a constant, ongoing controversy as to what a "healthy" diet is; I have enough opinion on that to write my own cookbook (I shall call it *Cooking with Buds*). There is solid evidence that a few specific foods are very damaging to the ECS (like processed sugar, artificial sweeteners, colors and flavors, as well as heated, refined seed oils). There are also several foods that are very healing to the ECS—either by introducing phytocannabinoids into the diet, healing endocannabinoid receptors, or by supporting/creating an environment for new endocannabinoid receptors to form, especially in our digestive system (hereafter referred to as our gut). This can be done by limiting inflammation, healing the gut microbiome, and consuming cannabinoids.

***"All disease begins in the gut." — Hippocrates***

The gut is a powerful system that can not only dictate our energy levels but also our mood and our body's ability to thrive and fight off diseases. It is heavily inundated with cannabinoid receptors, and they work together, along with the brain and liver, to form the gut-brain axis. We'll discuss how this important aspect of health connects it all in terms of stress, disease, movement, food, and supplements—tying in the benefits of cannabis and, more specifically, CBD.

*Keep in mind that with all herbs, adaptogens, and supplements, the qualities vary. Beware of added ingredients that may not be beneficial and could hinder the healing process, and know which part of the plant or fungi needs to be used to be effective. Many of these are not regulated. Please work with a clinical herbalist, naturopath, TCM practitioner, Ayurvedic practitioner, functional medicine practitioner, or integrative medicine practitioner to find the right method of use, type, and dosage that is beneficial for your condition. They will help you with the bigger picture, taking into consideration any pre-existing conditions, allergies or intolerances, and potential side effects.*

The gut consists of the digestive system, but when we refer to this, it also includes our "filtering" systems too—our livers, kidneys, and gallbladders included! All these parts and systems work together to process foods, drinks, medications, and supplements. They absorb nutrients, including vitamins and minerals, release hormones, filter out toxins, and eliminate waste, and are A MAJOR KEY to our foundational health.

Ideally, we would be buying, growing, or consuming foods that don't have or need a label, such as fresh fruits, vegetables, nuts, seeds, beans, and meats. They would be unprocessed, locally grown, in season, and untainted with chemicals, pesticides, and antibiotics. This is typically not realistic, however, for most of us.

Instead, it would be wise of us to, at a minimum, read and understand the labels. On ingredient lists in the U.S., it is required that the most abundant ingredient is listed first and then further listed in descending order from most to least. These labels help us discern whether or not a product is contributing to our health or detracting from it—merely providing calories and "keeping us alive."

Questions to ask are: Does it cause inflammation? Is it providing necessary vitamins, minerals, protein, and fiber? Is it feeding the "good" gut bacteria or the "bad"? Is it destroying or healing our endocannabinoid receptors and, in turn, preventing our immune system from doing its job?

Everything we consume has an effect on our body—either positive or negative. I would argue that there is no "neutral/neither," but there could be a "both."

*An example of a "both" might be carrot cake.*

***The "good"-***

- *Carrots provide beta-carotene (which converts to vitamin A, improving vision and immune function), fiber, vitamin K, potassium, and antioxidants.*
- *Nuts: healthy fats, protein, and fiber.*
- *Spices: Cinnamon and nutmeg are commonly used; they have powerful anti-inflammatory properties and can help with digestion.*

***The "bad"-***

- *Sugar causes an inflammatory response, weakens the immune system, enhances pain levels, spikes insulin levels (which can lead to insulin resistance), and can promote cancer cell growth.*
- *Frosting is typically made with sugar, butter, and cream cheese. It is high in calories, sodium, and saturated fat, with very minimal nutrients (tiny amounts of calcium, vitamin A, and protein found in the butter and cream cheese).*
- *Most commercial products are made with seed oils, artificial colors, and flavoring. Homemade is often best!*

The gut forms a strong bond, or a link referred to as an "axis," to both the brain and the liver. The connection between the gut-brain axis was observed and recorded back in 1765 by a Scottish physician. He noted that the gut possessed an abundance of nerve endings, which contributed to "nervous energy" throughout the body.

In recent years, though, the study of the gut-brain axis has been more publicized and researched, which has led to incredible advances in understanding more about our "second brain." This brain lives within the walls of our digestive system. This impacts everything—from how we view the connection between what we eat and our anxiety levels to how certain chemical additives, heavy metals, and lack of nutrient absorption can trigger autoimmune responses, diseases, and eventually lead to long-term health issues such as Alzheimer's and cancer.

I know that as research continues to define the connection between the brain and gut axis, Western medicine is finally supporting the idea that food equals fuel. Along with this, they are aligning with the fact that the quality of the food we eat not only supports energy levels and weight but can also be the key to preventing and (dare I say) curing diseases.

This also means the opposite is true. Low-quality foods, including toxic additives, can cause diseases as well. We hear about it every day—heart disease, diabetes, tooth decay, osteoporosis, and the list goes on.

These are not even the diseases that are predominantly caused by inflammation, though inflammation likely plays a part, which can be triggered by foods as well. As much as we'd all love to eat organic, healthy, balanced, and nutritious foods at every meal, it's not really feasible for all of us. Unfortunately, it can lead to unpleasant consequences that range from gassiness or bloating to issues such as irritable bowel syndrome (IBS) and "leaky gut."

Unhealthy eating, combined with stress, is a breeding ground for lifelong misery and the chronic conditions that stem from the unnecessary strain on our bodies. The inflammation alone, triggered by certain foods and drinks, can wreak havoc on our bodily systems. Gut inflammation has been linked to many serious issues, including seizures, anxiety, autism, eczema, and more.

There is a list, a mile long, of inflammatory foods (think anything with added sugar and most sugar alternatives, ultra-processed foods, and most "junk" foods). To make things even more complicated, some foods cause inflammation in certain people but not in others, due to intolerances, allergies, and even genetic predispositions. This is why it can be extremely valuable to work with a professional who can provide testing and guidance. Naturopaths, Integrative Health Practitioners, Holistic Clinical Nutritionists, TCM/Acupuncturists, Ayurvedic Medicine Practitioners, and Functional Medicine Doctors should all be well-versed in providing this kind of specialized care.

Our gut holds its own little world of organisms that allow digestion to happen, called a microbiome. What is a *microbiome*? It is the relationship between a microorganism and the body part that it lives in—in this case, bacteria within the digestive system. Within the gut, we need bacteria to help break down the food that we eat so that the nutrients are properly absorbed in our bodies. When these bacteria are out of balance, it can cause anything from mild discomfort and gas to cancer in extreme cases. Some bacteria are "good," and some bacteria are "bad." There are substances, molecules, and/or chemicals that feed bacteria and other substances that kill bacteria.

Most of us are familiar with antibiotics that kill bacteria. Many antibiotics are designed to kill specific strains of "bad" bacteria. However, others are more broad-spectrum and powerful and can unintentionally kill good bacteria along with the bad. This is why it is important to be aware of what we eat and take in. The things we eat and the medicines we take can either promote good bacterial growth or suppress it through the inflammatory process.

Prebiotics and probiotics found naturally in foods are a good way to help balance our gut microbiomes.

- Prebiotics promote the growth of good bacteria.
- Probiotics introduce additional good bacteria into our gut microbiome.

This "dream team" combination increases nutrient absorption and prevents disease!

As a bonus, probiotics can also help reduce stress and anxiety, further supporting the immune system and endocannabinoid system health. There are further studies linking the use of probiotics to improved cognition. Furthermore, research is being done to identify the impact of gut health on neurotransmitter production, such as increasing serotonin levels—a key chemical messenger that impacts everything from sexual function and appetite to blood clotting, happiness, and sleep.

You may be wondering, "How would cannabis fit in with all this?" CBD reduces stress and inflammation in the intestines AND helps balance out the microbiome within the gut. It both "feeds" the good gut bacteria and suppresses the over-production of the "bad" gut bacteria!

*Some other examples of foods that "feed" and support a healthy gut biome are:*

*Prebiotics:*

- *Peas*
- *Almonds*
- *Blueberries*
- *Garlic*
- *Asparagus*
- *Bananas*
- *Sourdough bread*

*Probiotics:*

- *Sauerkraut*
- *Kombucha*
- *Miso*
- *Kefir*
- *Pickles*
- *Kimchi*

*Yogurt is a popular choice for having probiotic benefits, but be careful because it is also often loaded with sugar, which feeds inflammation and causes it. Be cautious of ingredients when choosing your prebiotic and probiotic foods for gut health!*

Additionally, when you take prebiotics, it is shown to increase the number of cannabinoid receptors in our digestive systems, which improves the ability of CBD to control both healthy and unhealthy bacterial growth.

CBD can help promote healthy gut flora in three main ways:

1) Reducing overall inflammation.

2) Helping to control unhealthy bacterial growth within the digestive system.

3) Reducing stress and anxiety, which can lead to unhealthy eating habits.

A healthy endocannabinoid system is a strong combination of physical and mental health; both can be achieved through food, herbs, adaptogens, and supplements, in addition to the steps we covered in the previous chapter.

# CHAPTER FIFTEEN

# THC CAN BE RISKY BUSINESS

You may be wondering why supplementing with hemp and not medical or recreational cannabis. There are unique risks and rewards to using the various forms of cannabis. If you are learning about how to use cannabis as an alternative medicine or to self-medicate, these risks are important to be aware of. If you are utilizing hemp for preventative measures and for longevity, you should find this information very valuable. Pay extra attention if you or a loved one uses recreational cannabis regularly.

The high THC content in a vast majority of recreational cannabis comes with a lack of even more beneficial cannabinoids. It is grown predominantly for the "high" induced, and not necessarily for the long-term therapeutic effects in recreational cannabis dispensaries. Although there are terpenes and other beneficial plant constituents in all forms of cannabis, there are higher risks associated with the use of THC-dominant cultivars and products.

There are several major risks to frequent usage of THC products. These can include:

## 1. Tolerance

Over time, by ingesting THC in any form, your CB1 receptors, found in the brain, become reduced. This means that the same amount of THC won't give you the same effects—high or relief—the longer you use it. Instead of taking stronger or more frequent amounts in order to get the same sensations, it is suggested that you take a "reset break," allowing your receptor function to return to normal. This would mean abstaining from cannabis usage for a period of time, based on usage history and the strength of products being regularly consumed.

If you are a "new user" using regularly/daily for a year or less, you may need anywhere from two days - one week of abstaining to reduce your tolerance to a "normal-for-you" level. If the following list describes your usage, it may take a month or more to reset. Also, be sure to read the next section about addiction potential and cannabis use disorder.

- You have been a frequent consumer for many years.
- You predominantly take very strong forms of recreational cannabis, such as dabs and concentrates.
- You tend to keep cannabis in your system day and night.

## 2. Addiction Potential and Cannabis Disorders

Do you know anyone—it may even be you—who is addicted to the "runner's high"? As we mentioned in Chapter 10, the "runner's high" comes from the body releasing the endo-cannabinoid *anandamide* into the system by attaching to the CB1 receptors, giving you that euphoric feeling. Most runners live for experiencing that blissful reward for hitting a certain point in their running. It truly can be addictive!

Similar to anandamide, THC also attaches directly to the CB1 receptors in the brain, which gives people the "high" sensation experienced when using recreational and some-times medical cannabis. This sensation of a cannabis high, a.k.a. getting "stoned," can be addictive as well, as it triggers the same "reward center" in the brain.

As a huge cannabis fan, I am not against the use of THC. It has a special place in alternative medicine and is often a much safer alternative for numerous ailments than things that are commonly prescribed. Especially when it comes to pain, nausea, shrinking tumors, and muscle spasms, THC can bring relief without being as addictive or risky as opioids or other narcotics. Also, the risk of THC overdose is minuscule compared to that of traditional pain medications. With that being said, THC can be addictive.

According to Yale Medicine, "about 10% of people who begin smoking cannabis will become addicted, and 30% of current users meet the criteria for addiction." They also stated that "Synthetic cannabinoids, compounds manufactured to replicate individual chemicals found in cannabis, are much more potent than cannabis and therefore could be more dangerous."

Despite its addiction potential, there have been no deaths to date related to cannabis overdose. There are two conditions related to cannabis addiction: Cannabinoid Use Disorder (CUD) and Cannabinoid Hyperemesis Syndrome (CHS).

Cannabis Use Disorder (CUD) is the term used to describe cannabis addiction. It is classified as a psychiatric disorder since it can disrupt the user's life, their relationships, and their mental health. In Danielle Simone Brand's book *Weed Mom*, she addresses this disorder in depth. It is a great read and brings awareness to some topics rarely discussed, including cannabis addiction.

Many who struggle with this disorder experience cognitive difficulties, diminished social abilities, and even delusions. Some may even experience severe psychotic breaks as a result of heavy, ongoing usage (usually in conjunction with a mental health disorder). CUD is categorized based on severity, with DSM-1 being the least severe and DSM-5 being the most severe. This is diagnosed utilizing the CUDIT-R test, administered by a psychiatrist.

Current treatments include abstaining from usage, counseling, and cognitive behavioral therapy. Many European countries are even implementing the use of CBD in order to heal the endocannabinoid system for CUD patients. In a 2020 double-blind, randomized, placebo-controlled study,

CBD was 94% effective at reducing cravings for participants, meeting DSM-5 criteria after 4 weeks.

Cannabinoid Hyperemesis Syndrome (CHS) is a disorder resulting from long-term (years), heavy (daily or near-daily), and/or high-dosage cannabis use. It causes a lack of appetite, intense abdominal pain, frequent and severe vomiting, and nausea. It is more likely to occur if cannabis use began in the adolescent years. It can also be a sign of late-stage Cannabis Use Disorder.

The ONLY way to get rid of it is to stop cannabis (THC) use altogether. It will return if usage starts back up. Frequent hot baths, showers, and rehydration (including electrolytes) are necessary to ease the symptoms and find recovery. Newer treatments and research include the use of THC-free CBD. Recovery can take anywhere from 10 days to two months. During this time, it is important to re-strengthen the ECS and you can do this by utilizing the methods discussed in Chapter 13.

## 3. Psychoactive

Psychoactive products need to be used with extreme caution, regardless of legality. Safety is a MAJOR concern. Do not operate heavy machinery, drive, or be the sole care-giver of young children, babies, disabled persons, or others who may require you to drive or be fully alert and coherent under your care.

That being said, some users don't actually experience the

psychoactive effects of cannabis due to the body "absorbing" it into their deficient endocannabinoid systems. I know for a fact that there are MANY medical users who are more functional *while* using cannabis as medicine.

The effects are highly individualized. If you are a first-time or inexperienced user of THC products, be sure to proceed with caution. (See "Getting High Safely.")

Due to THC (as well as a few other cannabinoids in cannabis) being intoxicating, it is important to address the risk of maintaining sobriety for those who struggle with addiction.

As mentioned prior, THC can be addictive and can lead to Cannabis Use Disorder (CUD) and/or Cannabis Hyperemesis Syndrome (CHS). To avoid this, be sure to take "tolerance reset breaks", use lower percentage THC products (ideally 8-12%) and avoid concentrates (such as waxes, shatter, and live resins- most of which are vaped) and be sure to incorporate CBD and other healthy practices to keep your endocannabinoid system in balance-*especially if you are using for medical purposes*. There are exceptions to this suggestion, such as when using a live resin (known as Rick Simpson Oil, or RSO) as a life-saving cancer treatment or for other extenuating circumstances.

Utilizing cannabis remains a "gray" area for many who are recovering from substance abuse to other addictive, yet more dangerous, substances. Some recovery programs will allow cannabis as a "safer" alternative to opioids, cocaine, heroin, methamphetamines, and alcohol. A major reason for this is the fact that cannabis eases the cravings for these other addictive substances, even nicotine.

You may have heard the term "California sober" to refer to those who use weed but not alcohol or other drugs.

~or~

"Colorado Sober" refers to those who abstain from alcohol and other drugs except for cannabis and psychedelic drugs, like psilocybin (or magic mushrooms).

Although cannabis is a safe alternative for many, it is important to note that it is still a risky substance, especially for those who struggle with their mental health, which we will address in #4.

If you are in recovery or any substance abuse treatment program, I would highly suggest abstaining from using any THC products. It is SAFE to use CBD isolates, however, especially if you are subject to UAs. Please consult your treatment coordinator or other healthcare provider before utilizing cannabis products.

If substance abuse rehabilitation is a condition of probation or is court-ordered, it is highly likely that they will require you to abstain from cannabis use altogether. They will usually require regular, and sometimes random, urine analysis testing to provide proof of sobriety to the courts, counselors, probation officers, and other parties involved. (More on drug testing in #6).

## 4. Mental Health

Mental health has been at the forefront of many conversations lately, and for good reason. It is a topic that ranges from discussions about anxiety and depression to extreme scenarios—including school shootings and suicide.

In the past, this topic was usually discussed only behind closed doors. However, since 2020, and the extreme isolation, fear, and widespread generalized anxiety that the pandemic caused, mental health can no longer be ignored.

Prioritizing a healthy mindset, nurturing meaningful relationships, practicing stress management, and addressing as well as healing from trauma are all ways we ***should be*** preventing a decline in our mental health.

*~BUT~*

It is also proven that many mental illnesses can be genetic or inherited. Conditions such as Autism Spectrum Disorder (ASD), ADHD, schizophrenia, bipolar disorder, addiction, and depression all have genetic components.

These inherited genes put the person at a higher risk for developing these disorders later in life. This means that even though you may not exhibit any signs or symptoms of these disorders now, things can trigger these issues, such as traumatic events, unhealthy lifestyle choices, environmental toxins, injuries (especially head injuries), certain medications—including vaccines—and even chronic, unmanaged stress. *Super Genes* by Deepak Chopra, M.D., & Rudolph E. Tanzi Ph.D. is a great book that goes in depth on the human genome and optimizing your wellness despite these predispositions.

Mental health imbalances are VERY CLOSELY tied to addiction, whether it is through self-medicating for anxiety or utilizing substances to "fit in with the crowd." This can be linked to a lack of self-esteem, confidence, fear of rejection, and poor boundaries. Unaddressed, these issues can lead to depression and self-harm.

MANY large, high quality research studies confirm that the use of THC products could trigger latent (genetic or inherited) mental health disorders. This includes, but is not limited to: Schizophrenia, Bipolar Disorder, Tourette's, Obsessive Compulsive Disorder (OCD), and depression. This includes products that are hemp derived and only have .3% THC in them.

Over the years, I have counseled hundreds (possibly thousands) of people on the usage of cannabis products, frequently steering them toward hemp CBD products—specifically, ones without THC due to various risk factors associated with THC. You may (or may not) be surprised to hear about the number of people who don't want to try CBD products because "smoking weed" gave them so much anxiety. Maybe you had a similar experience. Even small amounts of THC—such as the amount in full-spectrum hemp products—can aggravate a person's anxiety and/or other psychological challenges, such as OCD, Tourette's, depression, and/or panic disorders.

On several occasions, I have been approached by post-combat U.S. veterans who have had medical cannabis prescribed or suggested to them by their healthcare provider. Although their provider was full of good intentions, the veteran/patient was not given much direction on what type of products to use (or not to use), only to be retraumatized by the THC triggering night terrors or episodes of Post-Traumatic Stress Disorder (PTSD) that they just can't shake. Using a CBD isolate product would have greatly helped these veterans without triggering the PTSD. With this new knowledge, they were VERY grateful once they made the switch.

In fact, **CBD has the opposite effect of THC when it comes to mental health.** It has been incredibly valuable as a complementary treatment for mental illness alongside cognitive behavioral therapy (CBT), counseling, and other lifestyle changes.

## 5. Growth, Development, and Reproduction Risks

According to a joint European research study done in 2020, "There is substantial evidence for a significant association between prenatal cannabis exposure and lower birth weight in offspring, and mixed results regarding later behavioural outcomes in the offspring. Adolescent cannabis use, especially heavy use, has been associated with altered executive function, depression, psychosis and use of other drugs later in life."

Since cannabis use is often compared to alcohol use (and underage drinking), it may be worth noting that heavy alcohol use has more severe, impairing effects both in the short term (through accidents and over-intoxication) and in the long term (through cancers, organ damage, and other associated diseases) than does heavy cannabis use.

It is also important to note that there are gender differences in the ways the body responds to cannabis. More research is necessary to reach an accurate conclusion about the long-term effects of adolescent usage and how it alters brain development over time.

## Men

Many studies confirm that frequent usage of THC leads to lower sperm count, low motility, and decreased sex drive. Keep in mind, however, that the higher occurrence of these male reproductive issues is associated with the co-usage of cannabis products AND cigarette smoking, alcohol usage, and/or additional illegal drugs. The results of THC use as a standalone substance and its impact on male fertility are inconclusive. There are many ongoing studies to learn more about this association.

One of the associations that is now coming to light is the connection between cannabis containing phytoestrogens, which can impair the natural hormone balance of biological males. Deeper research into this subject gives us additional insight, though.

* * *

*Phytoestrogens are natural compounds (discussed in Chapter 7: Flavonoids) that mimic estrogen—but not as strongly as the body's natural estrogen. Although it is primarily known as a female sex hormone, estrogen is also necessary for male sperm production, libido, bone health, mood, and brain function.*

* * *

A study done in March of 2020 explains that when gut bacteria lack certain microbes, the body reacts differently to phytoestrogens than it should, causing an issue with estrogen receptor activation in either low estrogen environments or high estrogen environments. Therefore, the impact is dependent on the male's baseline hormone levels. A high intake of certain phytoestrogens (such as the ones found in soy, flax, lentils, and hops) can be attributed to low testosterone levels.

While this has been seen in in vitro and in animal studies, the human studies have only shown minimal to no significant effect on testosterone when consumed in moderate amounts. Cannabis has a significantly lower amount of these types of phytoestrogens compared to the aforementioned plant products.

Phytoestrogens in cannabis will be highest when using a concentrated form of raw or full-spectrum product, such as resins, waxes, or shatter. There will be less in tinctures and edibles, and even less when smoking it in an unadulterated form. If this is of concern to you, an isolate-based product will remove ANY risk of consuming phytoestrogens in cannabis products—even with higher doses. As we learned in Chapter 8, all of the plant particles that would contain the phytoestrogens—the flavonoids, as well as the terpenes, waxes, lipids, and other cannabinoids—are removed and separated from the CBD during the remediation process.

Unfortunately, THC as a standalone cannabinoid, still carries risks outside of any potential phytoestrogen effects.

### Women

According to a study published in May 2022, titled, *Impact of Cannabinoids on Pregnancy, Reproductive Health and Offspring Outcomes*, there are a multitude of layers to consider regarding cannabis usage during pregnancy. Many studies were using NHPs (Non-Human Primates). When these studies were compared to human studies, there were a lot of conflicting outcomes.

It is also worth noting that in many of the human studies, the pregnant cannabis users shared many characteristics that could have affected the outcomes. These include being unmarried, younger, having a lower socioeconomic status, having lower education, or residing with a partner who also used or uses cannabis. It also mentioned that "women who use cannabis in polysubstance use with alcohol, tobacco, or other illicit drugs can result in an additive or synergistic effect." Keeping these things in mind, the following are some of the results found thus far…

Chronic THC exposure

Pregnancy and fetal outcomes:

- Preterm birth occurs due to THC passing through the placenta during gestation to the baby.
- THC found in breast milk during breastfeeding.
- Low birth weight
- Moderately increased risk of stillbirth.

The good news is that outside of pregnancy, cannabis products can actually be a great benefit for women of reproductive age, if they have no mental health risks and struggle with reproductive issues such as endometriosis, cysts, fibroids, painful menstruation, and/or ovulation—even with painful sex. THC binds directly to CB1 receptors, which are plentiful in a woman's reproductive system. Because CB1 receptors are closely tied to the sensation of pain, cannabis can be used to effectively treat menstrual and reproductive pain in women.

## 6. Career and School

Although this one doesn't apply to everyone, it is still worth considering if you are retired, unemployed, utilizing online schooling, working from home, or on disability. Two major career risks are based on safety (both in the workplace and safely arriving to and from the workplace) and drug testing.

First off, I don't condone driving while under the influence of any intoxicating cannabis products—either natural or synthetic.

In fact, I am including this as a career risk since many people drive or bike to work, and it can be dangerous to yourself and others to drive under the influence. DON'T DO IT!

There are some careers where using THC products presents a low risk, depending on the individual. Artists, creatives, many self-employed individuals, and those who work from home are just a few examples where it may be more "safe and acceptable" to be under the influence of THC while at work. There are some people (especially those who are medical-use patients) that work more effectively when intoxicated by THC, due to its ability to relieve pain, nausea, and other problematic symptoms of chronic illness. For these people, it is important to be mindful of transportation outside of career obligations. (I feel like *this* is what Uber Eats, Instacart, and DoorDash were created for!)

That being said, there are many jobs and careers out there that can become dangerous when you are high—because of the slower reaction time that many people present, because it can make you tired and therefore not as alert, and/or because it can hinder your short-term memory, focus, and concentration. Not only could you put yourself or others in danger, but you could also put yourself at risk for poor performance and the possibility of getting replaced by someone who does the job better.

The following is not an exhaustive list of jobs or careers that could be dangerous while intoxicated (there are many more):

- Anyone who operates heavy machinery—from backhoes to cranes, mining equipment, manufacturing plants, tractors, and even cement truck pumps.
- Those who utilize tools that cut, weld, drill, shoot, burn, or produce fire and/or electricity.
- Vehicle operators—pilots, drivers (CDL, Uber, pizza delivery, mail carriers, shuttle drivers), captains (ship, small boat, water taxis, cargo, ferry, fishing), and motorcycle operators (instructors, couriers, motocross riders, stunt performers)
- Jobs that require quick reaction time and/or accuracy include surgeons, dentists, veterinarians, nurses, firemen, linemen, EMTs, chefs, engineers, pharmacists, and professional and elite athletes.
- Anyone who works with chemicals and other dangerous substances.

Also important to note, there are many sober college campuses, collegiate sports, and high school athletic programs that prohibit the use of THC products. Sometimes the rules and regulations mention THC specifically, while others are more vague—prohibiting marijuana and other controlled substances.

Those who don't have to worry about transportation, school, or career risks, I would hope you are careful with the hobbies you pursue while under the influence of THC. I wouldn't suggest woodworking, blacksmithing, or rock climbing!

## On Drug Testing

Due to the inherent risks of cannabis intoxication, urine tests are commonplace in government jobs, the U.S. military, manufacturing jobs, professional athletics, healthcare jobs, and others. Some jobs will fire you immediately for failing a drug test, while others will offer a warning. Know the rules and requirements for your workplace.

These drug tests specifically test for THC and other controlled substances. This is usually done through urine analysis, or UA. (Yup, pee in a cup.) CBD does not have a urine test, but there are a lot of CBD products that contain THC and will test positive in a drug UA. Be mindful that broad-spectrum CBD products (that are THC-free) may also test as a false positive for THC, which we will discuss more in depth in the next chapter.

If you use or want to use cannabis in the workplace, but they require drug testing, it is suggested to use a hemp-derived CBD isolate product that has been 3rd party lab tested. This will ensure you produce a clean urine test (UA) every time, yet you will still enjoy the benefits of CBD and maintain workplace safety.

***All the above risks are not associated with CBD (without THC) product usage. We will cover what those options are in Chapter 17.***

## Legal

The risk of getting into legal trouble is dependent on where you live, based on local, state, and federal laws. There are some places in the U.S. where you can legally grow and consume your own plants, whereas in others, you may have to visit a dispensary or clinic. The legal age to partake in cannabis use in the states that allow recreational cannabis is 21 years old. This is only a risk in some states and countries. As of this writing in late 2025, the U.S. has 26 states, as well as the District of Columbia and Puerto Rico, that allow adult recreational-use cannabis (or have decriminalized it). A total of 41 states have legalized medical cannabis.

Cannabis reform is on the rise. Across the rest of the world, legalized (and decriminalized) countries include Canada, Mexico, Jamaica, Uruguay, Chile, Argentina, Portugal, Spain, Italy, Germany, Ireland, Belgium, Luxembourg, the Netherlands, Croatia, the Czech Republic, Georgia, Malta,

Israel, South Africa, Thailand, and the Australian Capital Territory. India allows some forms (sold by government-owned shops) only. Sri Lanka uses it in its traditional medical practices, as it has been part of its culture for centuries. There are some countries where all forms of cannabis (including THC free hemp CBD) are still illegal. These laws are constantly shifting, though, so be sure to look up current laws if considering usage abroad.

## CHAPTER SIXTEEN

# GETTING HIGH (SAFELY)

First and foremost, if you are under the age of 26 years or are pregnant or breastfeeding, and you are not working with a knowledgeable doctor or healthcare provider who specializes in the use of cannabis for medical conditions, it is NOT safe or recommended to use THC products (regardless of the legal age in many states being 21 years old). Hemp products have a low enough dosage (.3%) to give you the entourage effect for therapeutic usage of CBD products and will not get you high. If you reside in a state or country where THC use is not legal, I cannot condone usage in that state or country. Still not sure if you should do it? Please read the previous section on the major risks (***THC Can be Risky Business***) to frequent usage of THC products.

There are three important factors to consider for safe cannabis usage: product, dosage, and environment. These tips are good for both first-time and frequent consumers of internal-use cannabis products. The main routes for internal use are by mouth and inhalation. We will cover external use in a separate section.

Be aware that EVERYONE will have a different experience. Know that different methods of ingestion will vary in lengths of time to take effect and will last in your system for varying amounts of time.

1. Product testing, quality, and content (which we covered in Part 2)
2. Dosage—start low and go slow. This is common (good) advice given by budtenders and cannabis consultants everywhere! Know your method.
3. "Environment—safety is key!"

## Product and dosage: Common consumption methods

### Smoking

*Smoking* (joint, bong, blunt, preroll, pipe) involves lighting the cannabis on fire and inhaling the smoke in some form or another. It will typically take effect within 1 to 2 minutes. It may only take 1 to 2 "hits" to feel it, depending on your tolerance and the health of your endocannabinoid system.

*Fun fact: Just inhale and exhale—you don't have to hold the smoke in your lungs for any certain amount of time in order for it to work.*

The high may last up to 4 hours, but typically only lasts 1 to 3 hours. There are pros and cons to each of these methods of smoking. Some are more discreet and convenient, while others are smoother and more comfortable, yet not as portable. Filters may or may not be used. If you are not packing, rolling, or loading your own herb, use caution unless purchased from a reputable dispensary, as other herbs, chemicals, or substances can easily be added without your consent (known as "lacing"). Price, maintenance, and smoke quality also come into play with most methods.

Some people prefer smoking out of a bong in order to "trap" smoke/ash in the water so the smoke is more cleanly filtered and cooled as it enters the lungs.

## Vaping

*Vaping* (flower/bud/dry herb, liquids) instantly takes effect but wears off quickly, in general. It typically lasts 1 to 3 hours. Vaporizing cannabis can include the more common, portable, handheld vape "pens" or "carts"—short for cartridges. These can either be disposable or refillable.

Less common are the more expensive "home-use" tabletop vaporizers. Tabletop units are larger machines (about the size of a large essential oil diffuser) that typically come with a bag or tube(s). These bags or tubes are then filled with the vapor to be inhaled by a single person or individual tubes to be shared among friends.

Refillable vape pens consist of a rechargeable battery and a cartridge that may or may not be refillable. Some are designed to vaporize dry herb/bud that you can pack yourself—perfect for home growers and those who prefer to avoid residual solvents or additives.

Disposable vapes vary from single use to multiple uses until the built-in product inside runs out. Pre-filled vape cartridges are typically filled with liquids that are either oils, distillates, concentrates, or live resin. We'll go over those forms individually here:

- *Oils* is a vague term that can include a distillate blend of concentrated THC that may or may not include added terpenes (natural or artificial), carrier oils, and/or flavorings. Do your research on individual products; they vary greatly in strength as well as additives.
- *Distillates* are a product of processing and refining the plant in a way that concentrates a particular cannabinoid (in this case, THC) in a pure form. This increases the potency, typically 80-85% cannabinoids. It should specifically state the amount of THC per serving and/or per container in the case of vapes and other non-standardized dose types of products. This method tends to reduce the flavor and aroma since most of the terpenes, waxes, and flavonoids are filtered out during the refining process, as we learned in Chapter 9.

When not pre-packaged in vape carts, distillates can also be used sublingually. Distillates are sometimes "cut" with other oils or glycerides in order to produce a specific potency.

- *Concentrates* are similar to distillates, yet less refined in order to preserve the therapeutic terpene content. Concentrates may also include other cannabinoids. Forms of concentrates also include wax, shatter, budder, and crumble. These variances are due to the texture in the way that they are extracted and treated post-extraction. (For example, budder has a peanut butter-like consistency and is whipped in order to create a softer texture than the wax.)
- *Live resin* is a highly desirable form of concentrate made from flash-frozen cannabis in order to preserve the maximum amount of therapeutic cannabinoids and terpenes. It tends to have a very strong aroma, flavor profile, and potency.
- Vaping *flower, bud, or dry herb* is preferred for those looking for a "clean," discreet, and quick medicating method.

* * *

*Precautions for Vaping*

*Vape liquids-*

*Be aware that there can be fillers or cutting agents (vitamin E, MCT, PG, VG, S/S) that, when heated to a certain temperature, as in when vaped, can potentially cause harmful, even life-threatening side effects. Some effects are mild, such as nausea, but severe problems could include long-term respiratory issues known as "popcorn lung" and/or cancer. Also, use caution with any artificial flavors, terpenes, and fillers.*

*Vape Cartridges-*

*Harmful heavy metals from vaporizer battery coils are known to leach into the vape cartridges. This can cause heavy metal poisoning and other ill effects. Look for ceramic coils for a safer, longer-lasting product.*

* * *

## Sublingually

*Sublingual* means to take it (tinctures, oils, and oral syringes) and hold it under the tongue for 60 to 90 seconds so that it enters the bloodstream more rapidly through the mucous membranes. This allows for a quicker onset than edibles since it bypasses the secondary (stomach and intestinal) digestion. It only takes 5 to 15 minutes to "kick in" this way and is more bioavailable, meaning that a higher percentage of the product is absorbed and utilized as compared to some of the other methods (refer to the chart in part 3). The average effects for this method tend to be roughly 6 to 8 hours. The duration is typically shorter for men than for women. Things to note:

Typically, the "thinner" the product, the less concentrated it is. Oils, distillates, and concentrates can all be found in this thinner form. It is not uncommon for the tinctures to be alcohol-based, as this is how tinctures are traditionally made. However, some are made by blending a carrier oil or glycerin with the concentrate or distillate for ease of use and precise dosing. Keep in mind, though, cannabinoids are lipid (fat) soluble, which means that they need to bind to a fat in order to be fully absorbed by the body's ECS.

There is a HUGE variance of additives that can also be present—from flavorings (both natural or artificial) to terpenes, colorings, and preservatives. Always read your labels.

In this category, you may come across, or be recommended, oral syringes filled with Rick Simpson Oil (RSO), sometimes called FECO. They are highly concentrated and potent, often used as an alternative to or alongside cancer treatments. It is recommended that you work with a knowledgeable cannabis provider for dosing and usage with this type of product.

### Edibles

*Edibles* (candies, brownies, cookies, mints, THC-infused beverages, cannabutters, and more) offer practically endless options. BEWARE—these take the longest to kick in. Be patient. Give the product 45 to 90 minutes to take effect before opting to take a second dose. This method produces the longest-lasting effects, and you could potentially feel high for 6 to 12 hours.

Microdose: 1–2.5 mg THC

Standardized Dose: 5–10 mg THC

When taking edibles, your body actually gets high in two ways. As the THC makes contact with the liver, it breaks the THC chemical bonds and converts it into a metabolite called 11-hydroxy (OH)-THC. It then produces a secondary high, which reportedly can have an effect up to 4 times stronger than the THC itself! When your body metabolizes the edible, you will feel it in both your head (psychologically) and your body (physically). Keep in mind that everyone is different, so what one person experiences may or may not be what everyone else experiences, EVEN when consuming the same product.

A final note on both product and dosage: when CBD and THC are used together, they actually strengthen or enhance the effect, called the *"entourage effect." The entourage effect.* The entourage effect will actually increase BOTH the THC effects AND benefits of the CBD in medical cannabis, but you won't feel as "high" using both.

This includes using them separately but overlapping periods of effectiveness. For example, one could drink a CBD soda an hour before smoking a blunt, and you would feel the entourage effect immediately. The soda will take roughly 45 minutes to 1 hour to take effect; the blunt will be felt within a minute or two. This can be timed intentionally or not. Just be cautious of dosing when using them together. Use less than you think you may need or want, and build from there if desired. We will discuss the entourage effect and the pros and cons of it all in the next chapter when covering hemp usages and dosages.

## Environment

In order to enjoy medical or recreational cannabis responsibly in a safe and comfortable environment:

- Plan ahead so you don't have to go or drive anywhere.
- Unless under the care of a healthcare professional, avoid use while pregnant or breastfeeding.
- Avoid consumption around minors and keep products out of the reach of children.
- Be with responsible people whom you trust and with whom you are comfortable.
- Be sure to stock the area where you will be hanging out with a lot of healthy snacks, juices, plenty of water, and "creature comforts" such as soft blankets, pillows, music you enjoy, and possibly a journal or sketchbook in case you get "inspired" by any ideas that come your way.
- Pay attention to how you feel. Don't consume more than you "need" to. Again, go slow.
- Some people enjoy funny movies, videos, or board games, while others prefer coloring, meditating, napping, dancing, or just enjoying the company of those around them.

- If you prefer nature and can enjoy it safely, maybe you should sit outside in the fresh air.
- Some people prefer solitude, while others crave socialization. Sometimes, it just depends on the strain as well. Everyone is different in these preferences.

# PART IV

# THE ULTIMATE HEMP CBD GUIDE

DETERMINING THE TYPE, METHOD, AND AMOUNT FOR MAXIMIZING BENEFITS.

## CHAPTER SEVENTEEN

# SUPPLEMENTING WITH HEMP

Supplementing with hemp has become widely available in the U.S. since the passing of the Industrial Hemp Bill in 2018. The education surrounding the laws, benefits, risks, and safety profile of this incredible plant is far behind where it should be due to the unregulated nature of supplements in general. This makes it a challenge for both consumers and retailers. Once there is cannabis education more integrated into the industry on a sales/consumer level, the quality, reputation, and standards will improve, and the misinformation out there will decrease. When purchasing any of these products, it is important to understand how to read the CBD label.

In this next chapter, we will clarify the differences between the hemp products available on the market and what to look for in wellness products that are marketed as "CBD," "hemp extracts," and/or "hemp oils." It is also important to understand the terminology that is often listed on labels—typically misunderstood or confusing. We will explore the pros and cons of internal use vs. external use to help you understand the type of processing that the hemp underwent for extraction. We will also explore when, or if, it is appropriate to use each type to meet your goals.

There are many natural health practitioners, including chiropractors, naturopaths, integrative health practitioners, holistic health coaches, clinical herbalists, and doctors of TCM (Traditional Chinese Medicine), who are familiar with the appropriate uses of cannabis medicine. Some of the top medical schools in the U.S. are also finally getting on board with teaching about the endocannabinoid system; at a bare minimum, they are including the risks and benefits of pharmacological interactions, as well as the risks and adverse effects of THC-induced "cannabis use disorders." They are also including what type of cannabis product is appropriate for certain diseases, conditions, and disorders, which we began to discuss in Chapter 16.

More often than not, there are people who fall into one of two camps: the "naturalist" camp, where the idea is to keep as much of the plant unprocessed and intact as possible, preserving its natural healing properties, as with full-spectrum products. The other is the "purist" camp, where the goal is to have highly refined processing, with "reliable potency and dosing," such as with isolates or pharmaceutical-grade CBD. BOTH "camps" have very legitimate standings, and there are good arguments for using either one. It is a very personal decision that should be made when one is well-informed of the pros and cons of each type based on their individual circumstances.

If you live in a state with a longstanding and well-run

medical marijuana program, there will likely be many more reliable resources available to you. Unfortunately, many states are limited to a "doctor's note" that has a list of qualifying conditions, legal amounts to purchase and/or grow, a list of approved dispensaries, and limited information to provide regarding what to look for, the various methods of use (with pros and cons), what strains, and amounts to use for the specific condition.

Hemp CBD can be a much more accessible form of cannabis medicine that allows the public to utilize it for BOTH medical AND preventative purposes with an undeniable safety profile. Not only is hemp generally safe and non-toxic, but there is also no known lethal dose of hemp. Many forms of hemp have been utilized throughout history in cultures around the world with great success, often without fanfare.

## Hemp and CBD are often misunderstood.

There are many important things that should be known about hemp as a wellness product that help users understand what type of products might benefit them. There are three key factors to remember when you embark on your hemp wellness journey and several misconceptions that can deter people from using it in the first place. I hope this brings some clarity to the frustrations some experience when using hemp products for the first time.

### Key factor #1: *Hemp seeds and hemp seed products.*

As we discussed in Part 2, Chapter 6 in *Plant Anatomy*, hemp seeds don't have any THC, CBD or other cannabinoids. Hemp seeds are nutritious and have a great profile of omega fatty acids. These polyunsaturated fats are important to support brain health, eye health, and heart health. They are rich in omega-3s (ALA and stearidonic acid), omega-6s (linoleic acid and gamma-linoleic acid), as well as protein, fiber, and essential vitamins and minerals. Omega-3s have a mild anti-inflammatory effect, which is why foods like salmon, walnuts, and dark leafy vegetables, such as spinach, are listed on many "anti-inflammatory diet" lists.

- The seeds are a great addition to any diet and are touted as a superfood.
- Hemp milk is made by grinding the seeds into a flour, mixing it with water, and filtering out any solids. Again, it doesn't contain any CBD.
- Hemp seed oil is still made directly from the hemp seed by pressing and processing it, and it is used both as a cooking oil and a popular skin care ingredient. Since hemp seeds and hemp seed oil are rich in vitamin E, they are used in many popular lotions, cosmetics, and bath products to nourish the skin. With its nice absorbency and low comedogenic (pore-clogging) score, it is a healthy choice for moisturizing all skin types.

Hemp seeds, hemp milk, and hemp seed oil DO NOT, however, interact with the cannabinoid receptors like CBD does. *CBD* creates massive shifts in the body's endocannabinoid system in order to heal itself; *hemp seeds* don't, since they DO NOT CONTAIN CBD OR OTHER CANNABINOIDS. Remember "Hemp Myth #1" in Chapter 4? We discussed how there is NO CBD in hemp seed oil. Unfortunately, even as a topical, hemp seed oil doesn't have as many benefits as CBD for the skin and the tissues beneath, both functionally and cosmetically.

**Key factor #2: *Topical vs. Internal Use***

In order for hemp CBD products to create lasting, widespread, and systemic relief, they must be used internally, entering the bloodstream. There are a few products on the market that utilize chemicals that "break" the barrier, allowing the product applied to the skin to enter the bloodstream. These are often found in the form of a *transdermal* patch. Otherwise, if you aren't ingesting (eating or drinking) it, dropping it (under the tongue or in the eye), spraying (in the mouth or up the nose), inserting (such as a rectal or vaginal suppository), or inhaling (smoking or vaping) the cannabinoid products, they will provide only localized, short-term relief.

*Transdermal—relating* to, being in, or supplying a medication in a form for absorption through the skin into the bloodstream.

I am definitely not knocking all the amazing salves, balms, creams, serums, lotions, and massage oils out there! Topical CBD is used for:

- Wound healing (cuts, bites, and scratches)
- Skin irritation (abrasions, sunburns, and scrapes)
- Acne
- Hair growth
- Skincare (anti-aging, antioxidant, antibacterial, anti-inflammatory)
- Achy muscles—from overuse or post-workout.
- Joint pain - injury rehab
- Post-surgical pain and/or inflammation.
- Eczema rashes
- Arthritis pain
- "CBD topicals" also provide protection from infection due to their powerful antibacterial properties.

You will find that a growing number of massage therapists, estheticians, personal trainers, gym facilities, physical therapy offices, day spas, and even salons are utilizing the benefits of, and promoting, CBD topicals to enhance the results for their clients and patients. Topicals can come in many forms—creams, massage oils, bath salts, bath bombs, balms, salves, body butters, serums, roll-on gels, and ointments. They are all commonly sold, but not all are equally effective. In the next chapter, we will cover effective amounts of topical CBD to use for certain conditions and how long it may need to be used for optimal efficacy.

It is important to know that if you have an issue that starts on the inside and manifests externally, chances are you will experience much greater results from internal use—finding and addressing the root cause—than from external use, which frequently offers symptom relief while the root cause remains present.

That being said, only going "skin deep" can have its benefits too! I have heard countless people explain that they work for the government and can't use CBD products because they get random drug tested for THC. This would include all forms of military, postal workers, air traffic controllers, special agents, and so on. Although they get drug tested, they don't have to avoid ALL CBD products. Using CBD topicals and CBD isolates will not cause you to fail a drug test.

Topical products will not absorb into the bloodstream, so those who are using a CBD salve for achy joints or a CBD cream for eczema will not be at risk of getting fired from their government job (even with full-spectrum products that have a tiny bit of THC in them). I have had doctors, nurses, a DEA agent, firefighters, and police officers—all of whom use CBD regularly and get drug tested regularly—use quality CBD isolates, internally and/or topicals for pain and anxiety relief.

Many still don't want to risk it, and I don't blame them for not wanting to put their careers at risk, especially if they aren't sure if the topical has any *transdermal* properties. This is why it is important to know and understand the various forms of CBD that are on the market. Furthermore, it is important to find products with reputations you can trust and lab results to back that up. Can't risk CBD usage because of your job? Make sure you use a CBD isolate product; it completely eliminates all risk, even if used internally or the topical has transdermal properties. Which leads us to—

**Key factor #3: *Types of CBD Processing—full spectrum, broad spectrum, and isolates.***

Every type of processed cannabis product falls under one of these categories. The pros and cons of each fall to the individual using it. The division of these categories is more prevalent in the hemp industry due to the demand for therapeutic cannabis products that support the endocannabinoid system WITHOUT carrying the risks of THC usage (see what those risks are in Chapter 15).

The general breakdown looks like this:

***Full Spectrum***- minimal processing, .3% THC, CBD, minor cannabinoids, terpenes, flavonoids and other plant particles

***Broad Spectrum***- THC removed, CBD, minor cannabinoids, terpenes, flavonoids, and other plant particles.

***CBD Isolate***- 99%+ CBD (highly processed)

## CBD and Oxidative Stress

Regardless of what type of Hemp CBD product you would prefer, everyone can benefit from the internal use of CBD on a preventative level. As we age, the effects of oxidative stress build up in our bodies.

***CBD is a key to aging gracefully***

Oxidative stress, combatted by CBD's antioxidant property, is a great example of how CBD can help support the body from root cause issues. It also demonstrates how the body's systems are interconnected and how symptoms can arise, and be prevented, through lifestyle factors. Unfamiliar with oxidative stress or how it impacts one's body? Here's a brief rundown.

*Definition:*

Oxidative stress is a condition that occurs when there is an imbalance between free radicals (reactive oxygen species - ROS) and the body's ability to neutralize or detoxify them through antioxidants. Free radicals are molecules that contain oxygen and have an uneven number of electrons, which makes them highly reactive with other molecules.

*In Layman's Terms:*

Oxidative stress is like having too many bad guys, called free radicals, in your body and not enough good guys, called antioxidants, to stop them. Free radicals are unstable molecules that can cause damage to your cells—kind of like rust forming on metal or apples turning brown when left out.

Normally, your body uses multiple defense teams—one of them being the antioxidants—that fight these free radicals and keep everything in balance. However, when there are too many free radicals and not enough antioxidants, the bad guys can start harming your body, leading to problems like feeling sick or aging faster.

Things like unhealthy food and drinks, pollution (such as unclean air, perfumes, and artificial fragrances), or even heavy metals, microplastics, and EMFs can create more free radicals. To help your body stay strong, eating fruits and vegetables with lots of antioxidants can support your defense team!

Oxidative stress can be caused by external factors like pollution, radiation, cigarette smoke, and unhealthy diets, as well as internal factors such as inflammation or mitochondrial dysfunction. The body has a natural defense mechanism (e.g., enzymes and antioxidants like vitamin C, vitamin E, and glutathione) to counteract oxidative stress. If the balance is disrupted, free radicals accumulate, damaging cells, proteins, lipids, and DNA, which leads to various health problems. This cellular damage is linked to aging and many diseases, including:

- Cancer
- Cardiovascular diseases
- Diabetes
- Inflammatory diseases
- Neurodegenerative disorders (e.g., Alzheimer's, Parkinson's)

*So how does CBD combat oxidative stress?*

- It inhibits the production of free radicals.
- It inhibits the release of nitric oxide.
- It stabilizes free radicals by donating an electron to them, thereby preventing cellular damage.
- CBD negatively modulates A2A receptors, which dampens the harmful signaling that worsens oxidative stress and inflammation—especially in brain cells.
- Reduces inflammation—long-term inflammation leads to chronic disease.
- Boosts collagen production, which naturally wanes in the body beyond the mid-30s.
- Stimulates the immune system, protecting us from pathogens—viruses, bacteria, fungal infections, parasites, and more!

Using CBD, in effect, reverses the negative effects of oxidative stress and strengthens our body's defenses against repeated offenses. When CBD is used daily to prevent the damage caused by various external factors and to repair past damage done to our cell structure, we can effectively slow the aging process.

## CHAPTER EIGHTEEN

# WHICH CBD IS RIGHT FOR ME?

Finding the right type of cannabis product for you is highly individualized—your history, your preferences, the country and/or state you live in, your career, and your health goals all play a huge factor in deciding which wellness product will suit your needs. Ideally, everyone who sells CBD would be able to counsel the purchaser to the ideal product for them. Unfortunately, in the U.S. at least, the industry has grown so rapidly that once laws changed, education and research, to a certain extent, couldn't keep up with demand. These final chapters should give you plenty of information to get started on how to use cannabis smartly.

### Full Spectrum

You want the full benefits of THC without getting high?

Then Full Spectrum *Hemp* is your guy.

Hemp products with THC in them are considered full spectrum. If you remember from previous chapters, when hemp products are left in a more natural state there is typically a minimal amount of THC allowable during testing in order for it to qualify as hemp. This amount is UP TO .3% (dry weight). When purchasing dried flower/bud in any form, any packaging or information, on the product, should say the exact amount of THC that was stated in testing.

Full spectrum hemp products can be found in a dry flower form, which includes buds, joints, blunts, dry herb vapes, cones, and loose leaf teas. In this form of hemp, nothing has been removed from its original form (unprocessed). All the smokable forms of full spectrum hemp products still carry the risk of inhaling smoke, regardless of the benefits of the constituents. Some people "minimize" these risks by smoking through a water bong as a natural filter to prevent ash from entering the lungs. The dry herb vape still carries the risk of any chemicals/metals being burnt off the battery coil. The least risk of consuming the unprocessed forms is in drinking a tea, adding fresh or dried herbs into smoothies, juices, or foods, or infusing it into an oil or butter (cannabutter).

## Interesting Facts about Unprocessed Hemp

*Hemp in its natural form (unprocessed) has a very minimal amount of THC in it naturally- up to .3%. Even that small amount of THC, in hemp, "counts", when it comes to many of the risks, outside of the intoxication associated with THC use.*

*You'd have to smoke a LOT of hemp to consume enough to get "high" —think thousands of dollars' worth in a VERY short amount of time. However, even if you don't get high, you can still test positive for THC because it is fat-soluble and will stay in your system for an extended period of time.*

*It "looks" and smells just like other forms of cannabis, so many assume it will get you high. When grown for cannabinoid content—for CBD, CBG, CBN, or THC for example—the plants are grown and cultivated the same way, requiring the same nutrients, light, and pruning methods. Even experienced growers won't know the difference between high-THC cannabis and low-THC hemp plants just from the looks of them. They even smell the same, since they share the same terpenes! There ARE however BIG differences in hemp grown for fiber or seed than in hemp grown for cannabinoids.*

Full Spectrum Hemp *extract* is a vague term that describes the various forms that processed hemp comes in as a raw ingredient. Some examples of these are distillates, concentrates, and crude. Hemp goes through the same processes as recreational cannabis and medical cannabis to extract the active ingredients that were described in Chapter 8. In its "finished" form, the extract is typically diluted with a carrier oil or added to foods, drinks, and/or flavorings to provide a specific amount of cannabinoids per dose or per unit.

When hemp is distilled, infused, cooked, or processed into oils, tinctures (alcohol-based extractions), or edibles, without removing the THC through *remediation*, the product should state the amount of CBD—the total amount in the product and per serving—as well as include "full spectrum" somewhere on the label, or the ingredient list. It may be written as *full spectrum hemp extract," "hemp distillate," "whole plant formulation, full spectrum CBD oil, or occasionally just hemp oil.*

I will say it again, this is NOT to be confused with hemp *seed* oil, since hemp seed oil does not contain the beneficial cannabinoids you are seeking. There are MANY companies (we're talking about you, Amazon), that do not allow the sale of CBD products. This means that all the products that are being sold there that claim to have CBD in them are either mislabeled, or claiming that hemp seed oil has CBD in it. They are trying to claim that their hemp seed oil will help with anxiety, inflammation, and/or sleep, which are all benefits of CBD, and that is simply untrue.

The benefits of full-spectrum CBD oil are vast. The tiny amount of THC in a full-spectrum product allows the entourage effect to take place, as described at the end of Chapter 16. Cannabinoids, such as THC and CBD, when used together, have a more potent effect on the body. This holds true for cannabinoids interacting with terpenes, flavonoids, and other plant constituents as well. The entourage effect works in the context of both internal use and external use, but in different ways.

- Externally, the entourage effect allows for longer-lasting results, more pain relief, and deeper tissue penetration.
- Internally, it can amplify relaxation in order to help those with insomnia, increase pain relief, and improve appetite, nausea, and digestion.

*"Entourage Effect"* -- the effect of cannabinoids in combination with either each other and/or terpenes and flavonoids, in order to increase the therapeutic effects of each.

Pros: The entourage effect, individual benefits of the other plant parts, including the many benefits of THC without the intoxicating effects. The therapeutic effects can sometimes last longer, often at a lower dosage or amount used.

Cons: Even low THC levels can cause a positive drug test result with consistent use. Those with cannabis allergies can have a negative reaction. We know that THC can trigger latent psychiatric disorders, but also some minor cannabinoids (notably CBN) can aggravate mental health conditions too, which include anxiety and Post-Traumatic Stress Disorder (PTSD), two common conditions CBD is used to relieve. It is also less safe for children and ***unsafe*** for pets, regardless of what is being sold in many pet stores.

## The THC and CBD Comparison: Hot Topics

It has been interesting to see where the separation between CBD and THC really comes into play. Prior to 2018, much of the research on CBD was viewed through the lens of "Marijuana vs. Medical Marijuana," comparing solely THC vs. THC + CBD combinations. Once researchers started studying CBD as a singular compound (an isolate), the studies revealed some fascinating findings, especially among some of the hot topic conversions of today.

- Immunity. CBD can act as an *immunomodulator,* which means that CBD can *stimulate or suppress* the immune system based on the body's needs. THC, on the other hand, tends to be an immunosuppressant, which is great if you have an *overactive* immune system, but not if you have a weakened one. This can mean the difference between being more susceptible to a disease, virus, or other pathology when using THC products versus being protected against it by using CBD!
- CBD can help with weight management. While THC is known to stimulate the appetite, CBD is known to reduce appetite and cravings—especially when those are fueled by stress or emotions. It also lowers cortisol levels and promotes the conversion of white fat, which stores energy, to brown fat, which burns energy. Better sleep quality, which is often experienced with CBD, is linked to healthy weight management as well.
- Addiction and tolerance have always been debated topics in cannabis conversations. THC connects to the CB1 receptors; therefore, there is a strong link to the reward and addiction pathways. It is an *agonist* to these receptors, meaning that it directly activates them. HEAVY THC use (low to moderate amounts at a young age, or heavy/intense usage over a shorter period of time) can lead to changes in these receptors, resulting in a higher tolerance

and eventually making one more prone to addiction.

In contrast, CBD doesn't DIRECTLY interact with the CB1 receptors, so it doesn't have the same effect on the reward pathways that THC does. A 2021 review, "Role of Cannabidiol in the Therapeutic Intervention for Substance Use Disorders," shows promise in the reduction of drug-seeking behaviors. It also demonstrates the ability to alleviate withdrawal symptoms by modulating multiple neurobiological systems and exhibits no abuse potential. The substances in the study included nicotine, cannabis (THC—cannabis use disorder), alcohol, opioids, and psychostimulants, such as cocaine and methamphetamines. The study included both animals and humans. While more long-term human studies are needed for the psychostimulant category, all the other categories showed reductions in use, cravings, anxiety, withdrawal symptoms, and improved treatment retention while being treated with CBD. Moreover, it is typical for CBD users to need LESS CBD over time to achieve the desired effect on the body, as opposed to building a tolerance and needing more. CBD is currently being utilized for addiction recovery worldwide due to its safety profile and efficacy in case studies.

- Memory: You may be familiar with the stereotype of "stoners" having short-term memory loss. While THC impairs memory, CBD once again has the opposite effect. Individual responses may vary and be dose-dependent. Co-usage in medical cannabis products can vary based on the CBD:THC ratios, and this typically has short-term effects for both THC-only products and products that contain both.

## Broad Spectrum CBD

An opportunity to glean all the benefits of CBD without incurring the same risks of THC is by using a *broad-spectrum* CBD product. The label will likely either say "Broad Spectrum" directly on it, "THC Free" distillate, or "THC Free" hemp extract. If it only says "THC Free," it could be either broad-spectrum or CBD isolate, so you will have to read the label further for more details to find cannabinoid content or see if it says "extract" or "distillate" on the ingredients list. If it doesn't, it's likely a CBD isolate product.

*Broad Spectrum Hemp* is a whole plant extract; THC is removed from the extract, leaving behind CBD and other cannabinoids, terpenes, flavonoids and other natural plant constituents. Broad Spectrum starts in distillate form to be added as an ingredient to make a variety of products for both internal and external use. It is similar in appearance and scent to full spectrum extract.

This form allows the user the benefit of the "entourage effect" for increased pain relief without THC as a risk.* Like with full-spectrum products, you will benefit from the therapeutic properties of all the plant components working synergistically.

* It is important to note that Cannabinol (CBN) is a minor cannabinoid that can be found in any cannabis or hemp product and can frequently be found in broad-spectrum hemp products. CBN is formed by the degradation of THC. As THC ages or is exposed to mild heat or light over time, it loses a molecular bond, thus forming CBN. This can lead to three things:

1. It can test "false positive" for THC drug tests (think of the "poppy seed muffin" effect).
2. It shares many similar benefits and risks as THC such as helping with sleep, but it can also aggravate anxiety, PTSD, bipolar disorders, and other mental health conditions.
3. It can be mildly psychoactive. This may be a challenge for those looking to overcome addiction by steering clear of intoxicating substances.

It is important to see lab test results or find out the types of minor cannabinoids in your broad-spectrum product if these risks are a concern to you, especially if you are a regular, consistent consumer.

Both full spectrum and broad spectrum hemp products taste and smell "hempy" because of their more natural, often less processed form. These two processing levels can be "certified" organic, giving the consumer some peace of mind that they are ingesting or applying a clean and natural product to their bodies. This is especially important for those who strive to steer clear of pesticides and other contaminants. Another THC-free alternative is using a CBD isolate.

## CBD Isolate

CBD Isolates get a bad rap. Although they are a THC free alternative to Broad Spectrum and were an isolated cannabinoid since 1940, they are still often misunderstood and misrepresented. Chapter 8 explained how individual cannabinoids can be extracted out of the distillate (the hemp or cannabis extract in its concentrated form). This is how "pharmaceutical grade" CBD is made - such as the seizure medication *Epidiolex*. In this form, CBD is an off-white powder, and gets mixed with a carrier oil in order to be absorbable by the body. CBD Isolate products carry NONE of the risks of a full spectrum. Since CBD isolate is just pure cannabinoid (99%+) it is easy to formulate with, easy to use, consistent to dose, and carries less risk and side effects as the more "hempy", smelling counterparts. I like it because of its purity and the fact that it's more consistent when finding, tracking and controlling the dosage of CBD that works for you.

*For example:*

A 1 oz (30 ml) dropper bottle of CBD Isolate tincture that is labeled 1500 mg CBD will have 50 mg of CBD per 1 ml dropperful (one serving) every time.

On the other hand,

1 oz (30 ml) dropper bottle of Full Spectrum Hemp Extract may have 22 mg CBD per serving in one batch, but in another batch, it may have 26 mg CBD per serving (with varying types and concentrations of other minor cannabinoids per batch). The bottle will still likely say 60 mg Hemp Extract per serving (which is still accurate), but the composition from batch to batch can vary. This occurs not only between brands but also often within brands as well.

This doesn't mean that the quality is poor or that the product is bad; it is just the nature of using a product filled with natural constituents. This is much like any herb in the supplement industry.

Thankfully, CBD is VERY forgiving to work with, so it may not be a big deal to most people, but for people like me, I know that if I have a little bit more than my "sweet spot" for dosing, I can get a bit lethargic. Some days, I need all the energy I can muster! I love the predictability of an isolate, especially for daytime use.

This also means:

1. There is no entourage effect when using it. You aren't getting the individual benefits of the terpenes, so it may not seem as effective at first.
2. There will be clean drug tests and no concerns that CBN may cause a false positive, as with many broad-spectrum products.

3. It also means that without the other plant compounds present, the dosage must be higher in order to have the same effect. It may also not last as long in the system.

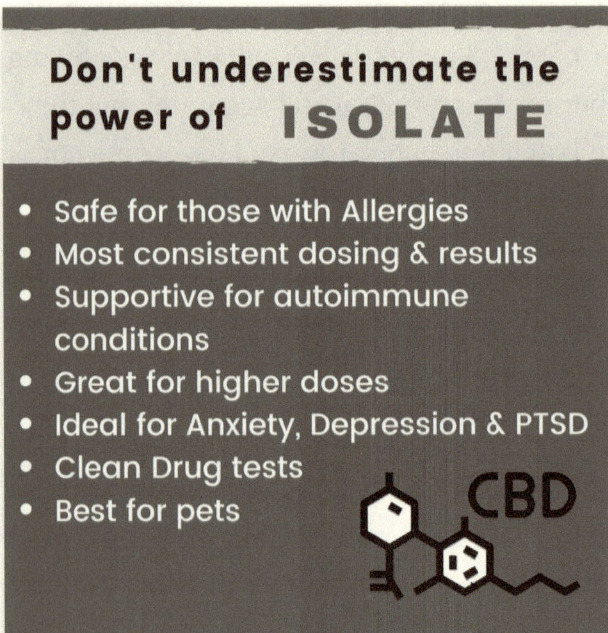


There is a LOT of misinformation and confusion about CBD isolates. CBD isolates can be very powerful, but because of the way they lack hemp smell, taste, and color, people assume they are an inferior form of CBD and don't give them a chance. On top of that, CBD *can be, but isn't always,* created in a lab, and unfortunately, ***lab-synthesized CBD*** commonly has more "side effects" than naturally extracted CBD does. That means that when companies are trying to sell you their "natural, whole-plant extract" and are trying to convince you that isolates have more side effects, it is because of the "side effects" they read about in the research studies—many of which were synthetic forms of isolate.

Prior to 2018, the research on isolates had primarily focused on pharmaceutical usage and extreme doses. That being said, lab-synthesized CBD is predominantly used in research settings. Most cannabinoid research studies are funded either by the government, universities, the NIH (National Institutes of Health), the NIDA (National Institute on Drug Abuse), or private companies. Recent legislation has opened the doors to expand the research, allowing larger studies to overturn some of the previously held beliefs that we now know are inaccurate.

Occasionally, companies will add the words "terpene enriched" or "added terpenes" if they have enhanced the CBD isolate product to include the therapeutic benefits of terpenes. This makes it more similar to a broad-spectrum product since the added terpenes create the entourage effect, without any risk of false positive drug tests or triggering any mental health challenges—the best of both worlds.

## CHAPTER NINETEEN

# BENEFITS, DOSING, AND THE LIFE-CHANGING STORY OF CBD

There are 4 main "anti" properties that CBD holds, contributing to its unique and powerful healing benefits: anti-inflammatory, antioxidant, antiseizure, and antianxiety. In addition to a multitude of other important benefits, it can make an impact on those with both short-term injuries and chronic conditions.

As seen in the chart on pg. 78, there are 18 healing properties of CBD listed. One "healing property" can benefit multiple diseases, disorders, and conditions. Inflammation is the root of any "-itis" condition—from arthritis to gingivitis to bronchitis to meningitis—as well as many conditions (for example, diabetes) that have multiple "symptoms" that CBD can help manage. Using diabetes as the example, CBD can help balance blood sugar levels as well as prevent peripheral neuropathy (numbness in the extremities) through CBD's neuroprotective benefits.

Sometimes CBD addresses "root-factor" causes, while other times it merely helps to manage the symptoms. By understanding CBD's role in the ECS, we can put together the pieces of the puzzle regarding how disease begins in the first place, how to prevent it, and how to make shifts in our daily lives in order to prevent many of the issues from which we seek relief.

CBD can be used like a daily supplement for general wellness to manage everyday stress, but many people use it for various other purposes. There is A LOT more research being done on this subject, and current scientific research, case studies, and anecdotal evidence—both in the U.S. and abroad—have illuminated a huge range of benefits for various conditions when used internally, including, but not limited to:

- Neurological disorders and conditions (such as epilepsy, multiple sclerosis, ALS, Parkinson's disease, Huntington's chorea, stroke, Alzheimer's disease, dementia, nerve damage, traumatic brain injuries, and migraines)
- Pain and inflammatory conditions (arthritis—both osteoarthritis and rheumatoid arthritis, bursitis, degenerative disc disease, post-surgical pain, tendonitis, autoimmune diseases)
- Neuropsychiatric illnesses (anxiety, depression, PTSD, autism, ADHD, OCD, and alcoholism/addiction)
- Gut and metabolic disorders (diabetes, obesity, colitis, Crohn's disease, IBS)
- Reproductive and endocrine conditions (endometriosis, some forms of reproductive cancers, PCOS, PMS, perimenopause and

menopause, fibromyalgia, which is also considered neurological, and thyroid disorders)

- Skin diseases (acne, dermatitis, psoriasis, eczema, and rosacea)

**Benefits for Specific Conditions**

(F)ull Spectrum (B)road Spectrum (I)solate

| | | | |
|---|---|---|---|
| FBI | Stress Relief | FBI | ALS |
| FBI | Inflammation | FBI | Acne |
| FBI | Nerve Pain | BI | Addiction Recovery |
| FBI | Alzheimer's | BI | Autism |
| FBI | Parkinson's | I | ADHD |
| FBI | Arthritis | FBI | Spinal Cord Injuries |
| FB | Nausea | FBI | TBI |
| FBI | Spasms | F | Tumor Reduction |
| F | Migraines | I | Immune Support |
| F | Fibromyalgia | I | Social Anxiety Disorder |
| FBI | Multiple Sclerosis | I | Weight Management |
| FBI | Pain | I | Depression |
| I | Panic Disorder | FBI | Seizures |
| I | PTSD | I | Asthma |
| I | Generalized Anxiety | I | Depression |
| FBI | Endocrine Balance | I | Libido |
| I | Schizophrenia | | |

There are many studies and a lot of promise in the research currently being done regarding its effectiveness against antibiotic-resistant bacterial strains (such as MRSA). Even though CBD is not technically a sedative, it is not uncommon for people to use it for longer, deeper sleep, as it can help people relax, calm the mind, and relieve stress. In higher doses, it can cause a bit of drowsiness, which can be considered a possible side effect. Typically, if it is making you drowsy, you are just above your "sweet spot" dosage-wise, unless you are using it for insomnia, of course.

CBD is an incredible molecule that our bodies were designed to interact with. You don't have to be "sick/unhealthy" to benefit from CBD use. CBD use can be a PROACTIVE way to stay healthy and age gracefully. Keep in mind that CBD is only one tool in your toolbox, and although it can be a catalyst for MANY positive changes, it is NOT the only thing that you will need in order to achieve your health and wellness goals. This chapter is wholly devoted to that topic and should clarify who would benefit from it. Mostly, it will demonstrate how to use it effectively and what changes in your body you can expect from long-term usage. I'd like to set the stage for this by sharing a very personal account.

Like many of those who have had life-changing experiences that changed the trajectory of their future, I had an "awakening" that truly changed my life a few years back. I have always been somewhat of an "open book" when it comes to sharing my experiences—both successes AND failures. Since I believe that we were all put here on this earth to help each other grow, learn, love, and connect—both with each other and our higher power. I believe that God has a plan for us all, and that if we have faith and give the glory to HIM, by following His calling for our lives, He will bless us eternally. Whether you believe this or not is up to you.

## How "CBD Isolate" Changed My Life

It was August of 2018. If you have been following my timeline up to this point, I was just over four years into my CBD journey—researching, formulating, retailing, wholesaling, and educating about CBD as fifteen years into my massage practice. I had a small clinic in North Idaho, Northwest Medical Massage, that employed four hard-working people who were integral in contributing to the thriving practice that predominantly served a clientele seeking rehabilitative therapies for their chronic pain, athletic injuries, or mobility challenges. We offered cupping therapy, myofascial release, sports massage, prenatal massage, as well as CBD massage, of course. My husband and I were in Las Vegas so I could attend the World Massage Festival for the second time.

Once the four-day conference was over, my husband and I gave ourselves an extra couple of days to have fun. On our way to breakfast on one of the final mornings, we headed up a long, wide, and open flight of stairs in our casino hotel when my heart and stomach sank as I collapsed to the floor. My husband caught my full weight before I could tumble down. Concerned, still holding me up, he asked, "What's going on?"

Crying, I whimpered, "I can't feel my legs."

Lovingly and instinctively, he scooped me into his arms and carried me up the flight of stairs to the bench at the top. On the way up, he asked, "Can you move your feet?"

Shaking and terrified, I whispered, "No."

He gingerly sat me on the bench at the top. Only seconds later, which felt like forever, I heaved a HUGE sigh of relief. "I can feel them again! It's coming back."

I rotated my ankles, wiggled my toes, and extended my legs, but I didn't quite trust myself to stand still. It had only been a minute or two of paralysis, but it was the wake-up call I obviously needed.

"We need to get you to the doctor to talk to her about your health issues." I finally agreed.

My symptoms had been piling up over the previous few years. Sure, I knew I had some long-term damage from some of my past injuries—car accidents, dislocations, and falls. Some of the things I was experiencing—the fatigue, the body aches, anxiety, the hair loss, the insomnia—I chalked up to perimenopause. However, I still had questions and concerns.

Why was my digestion so off?

Why did I have bouts of weakness in my extremities?

Why did every single joint in my body hurt ALL the time—especially when it was cold, or stormy, or if I even exercised a little bit?

Why did I start forgetting simple things that used to be second nature to me (like using the cruise control in the car or how to get to my parents' house, which is only 8 minutes away from me and has been for the past 20 years)?

Why did I feel like there was something wrong with me that I just couldn't explain?

The first few appointments with my doctor went about the

way I would have expected—tests, followed by blood work and then more tests. Referrals to several specialists—Rheumatology to begin with. Blood work showed extremely high levels of inflammation, but everything else looked "within normal range." This is with the exception of hypothyroidism, which I had known about and been treating for several years prior. It was the only medication I was on at that point. It was a process of elimination while I waited for months to get into the rheumatologist. MS? Nope. Lupus? Nope. Rheumatoid arthritis? Nope. I was frustrated. I led a pretty healthy and active lifestyle. I hiked, rode bikes with my kids, golfed, did yoga, didn't drink a lot, didn't smoke, ate clean, took vitamins, prioritized sleep, and had a good relationship with my family and friends—why did I feel *so awful*?

My doctor, whom I really respect, mentioned going on the anti-inflammatory diet while I waited to get into the rheumatologist. She also offered me pain meds, which I politely declined; corticosteroids, which made me SUPER sick for three days straight before I gave up on them; and gabapentin (an anti-seizure medicine that is also often used for nerve pain, and sometimes sleep and anxiety). The gabapentin made my dizziness and nausea worse, yet still didn't do much for the nerve pain I felt intermittently.

I was all about the anti-inflammatory diet idea, but I had already been on it for the past three years. Although I would continue, I definitely needed something else. I continued working through all this but was gradually cutting back my hours in order to accommodate medical appointments and hopefully allow my body to heal a bit. Despite working less, the symptoms continued to progress. Sometimes, one arm and hand would go completely numb from the shoulder down during a massage session. I came close to fainting during sessions a couple of times; telling my client, "Sorry, I have to stop for a minute and lay on the floor and put my legs up a wall," didn't feel too professional.

Over the next few months, I prayed hard for help and answers and came to realize two things.

1. I should practice what I preach. If my family or friends were going through what I was, and they knew their inflammation levels were that high, they had nerve and digestive issues, along with widespread pain and anxiety, I would suggest taking CBD. I hadn't been. Crazy, right? Sure, I would use the topicals on my sore joints and the facial serum for the youthful glow it gave me, BUT from then on, I would treat myself *the way I would advise them: find* my ideal dose and be consistent. Include supportive habits: prayer, sunlight, vitamin C, turmeric, breathwork, gratitude, gentle movement, slowing down, accepting help, and protecting my energy.
2. I needed to stop doing massage, even if it was just until I got my health issues under control. This was easier said than done, but I had my husband and family's full support and encouragement. I know

> that I am so blessed and grateful that this would not be a big financial burden on our family. My employees and clients were extremely understanding and wondered why I didn't shut down sooner. Not everyone has this privilege, I know, but I mourned the loss like an old friend. It was my passion and my purpose, and I had to say goodbye.

I shut down my massage practice in December and started to implement the "new" practices before my rheumatology appointment in mid-March. By Christmas, my condition had worsened to the point where I couldn't leave my bedroom and bathroom most days of the week. My husband had to frequently carry me up the stairs of our home if I felt well and ambitious enough to make it into the kitchen downstairs that day. My kids helped me walk when I was too weak or dizzy to go to the living room for a change of scenery.

My gut was so bloated it looked like I was five months pregnant! I would have constant pain in my gallbladder area, on top of all the other digestive distress and pains that I was always experiencing. During the roughest months, my pain levels hovered around seven to eight on the pain scale. "Mind over matter," I reminded myself. "The pain is not that bad, and it could always be worse" became my mantra. Just breathe; it WILL get better. I continued using CBD isolate tincture 2 to 4 times a day consistently and practiced those supportive habits to the best of my ability.

By mid-January, my pain was getting less and less. Any peripheral neuropathy (numbness and tingling in the extremities) that I had been experiencing was slowly subsiding. I was starting to sleep better, and my bowel habits were improving. I got the call that the rheumatologist had a cancellation and could see me "early" in February.

By the first week of February, my pain levels had dropped to a consistent 4 on the pain scale. I was elated, even though I still had a lot of issues I was contending with. While in the waiting area at the rheumatology office, I noticed the staff photos on the wall that showed there was a naturopathic rheumatologist on staff as well. Intrigued, when the doctor called me in, I asked if there was any way the Naturopathic Rheumatologist could join us as well since there was a good chance my body typically didn't tolerate prescriptions well. He joined us.

Two major things happened at that appointment. The first thing they did was order more blood work to see if my inflammation levels were still super high. They rushed the results so we could compare them right there, on the spot. He was shocked. He showed me the first results from my general practitioner in August. My CRP levels, which measure C-reactive protein, an inflammation marker, were in the 60s (anything over 10 is a concern). By the appointment with him in February, the inflammation levels were nearly non-existent. He asked what I had changed during the months I had been waiting. I told him about adding internal-use CBD and the supportive habits I had been practicing more consistently. He was shocked and impressed by the results. Being a Washington State practitioner, he was well aware of the impact medical cannabis had on chronic pain. However, when I mentioned that I was using CBD isolate, he couldn't believe it. The numbers were clear as day.

After a long discussion of my health history, symptoms, blood work, test results, and medical records, we were able to eliminate several more diseases, syndromes, and conditions that didn't fit. The things that did fit, however, were:

- Ehlers-Danlos Syndrome, a.k.a. EDS (Type 4, Hypermobile)
- Widespread osteoarthritis
- Centralized sensitization
- Dysautonomia
- Likely mast cell activation disorder
- IBS
- Potential POTS

Due to the nature of some of these issues, I was referred to a cardiologist, a GI doctor, a geneticist, and an immunologist. With those visits, we also discovered my mild gastroparesis (delayed stomach emptying), hyperkinetic (overachieving) gallbladder, and MTHFR gene mutation. I did not have POTS, but I have bradycardia, which explained the many hospital visits I had as a child due to fainting.

As scary as having all these conditions sounded, I was RELIEVED. I wasn't going crazy. The pain wasn't in my head. Even though I looked like a woman in her late 30s, my insides told a different story. One of the practitioners mentioned it looked like I had the joints and organs of an 80-year-old. With these answers, I had something I could work toward. EDS is a genetic collagen disorder. It is where one's body forms connective tissues that are overly stretchy due to defective collagen. It's flexible in a way that can be damaging to joints, organs, blood vessels, and even nerves. Because collagen makes up the coating that surrounds and encases both small and large structures, it can cause a variety of issues in the body. The weakness in the collagen matrix can lead to missed synapses (from brain fog to spontaneous paralysis), easy bruising, slow wound healing, a stomach and intestines that don't contract as well as they should to push food through, to keep hip bones in the socket (and many issues in between). My body was deteriorating quickly, from the inside out.

I learned a lot about my body and how it was supposed to function versus how it was ACTUALLY functioning. Learning all about these conditions, what causes them, how to prevent and/or treat them, and what type of lifestyle changes can make a positive impact on daily quality of life has been so helpful. This is not only for my own journey but also for the purpose of coaching others who struggle with similar chronic conditions.

While writing this book, it has now been seven years since "the scare" in Vegas. I thank God for showing me that my pain can be turned into a new sense of purpose. I try not to dwell on the things I can no longer do. I am back to riding bikes with my kids, golfing, hiking, and I have even eased myself into working again—teaching pathology and business classes at our local massage school while teaching CBD workshops on the side. I have also had the privilege and honor of sharing my inspirational story and stage with some incredible motivational speakers and providing coaching on a case-by-case basis.

I am so grateful that my pain levels typically hover around a 2-3 on the pain scale in cold winter weather, or a 1 on the pain scale in warm weather. I still take CBD almost daily, but at a significantly lower "maintenance dose" than when I started. I no longer need to take thyroid medications, as it is now well regulated since using CBD consistently. No more peripheral neuropathy. My IBS is no longer an issue. My anxiety rarely crops up anymore. No more distended gut. No gallbladder pain. I consume extra sodium to manage my low blood pressure. Lion's Mane works wonders for brain fog, focus, and memory issues. Pilates has become my friend.

I have gotten better at listening to my body, and my faith is SO MUCH stronger - HE is the only true healer. I try to move my body and get sunshine daily; I will forever be grateful for my support system that got me through that rough spot on my journey and continually has my back. I hope my story inspires people to seek the one true healer—

Jesus Christ—and to share the hope, love, and light HE has for us all. Yes, God created cannabis, but it is just a tool. A tool to connect, share, start the healing journey, and hopefully open your eyes to new possibilities and maybe even a new sense of purpose and renewed faith, like it has for me.

## CHAPTER TWENTY

# YOUR GUIDE TO HEMP CBD

At this point, you should be pretty familiar with the benefits of CBD. You may even be a seasoned user or have only tried it a time or two and weren't sure if it even works. You can buy it practically anywhere. Chances are, though, you may not have had any opportunity to learn HOW to use it in order to have lasting, effective results.

This guide is written not only for the everyday consumer but also for those who are providing these products to the consumers—consultants, sales reps, growers, distributors, retailers, caregivers, healthcare providers, wellness clinics, supplement stores, alternative medicine practitioners, manufacturers, formulators, and yes—even doctors.

So how do you get started using CBD? Let's clarify some things first. In some states where medical cannabis and/or recreational cannabis is legal, the products may have a "higher than the legal limit" of THC for a hemp product, which actually just puts them in the medical cannabis category. They have their own rules for labeling and/or testing and may or may not contain CBD.

This usage guide *does not* apply to those products. It only applies to products that DO NOT CONTAIN more than .3% THC dry weight-classifying it as HEMP which is federally legal under the 2018 Farm Bill.

Those things being said, let's dive in to determine what type and how much CBD will help you reach your wellness goals. Assuming all hemp products are legal and available in your area, we would start by determining if you need an external-use product, an internal-use product, or both.

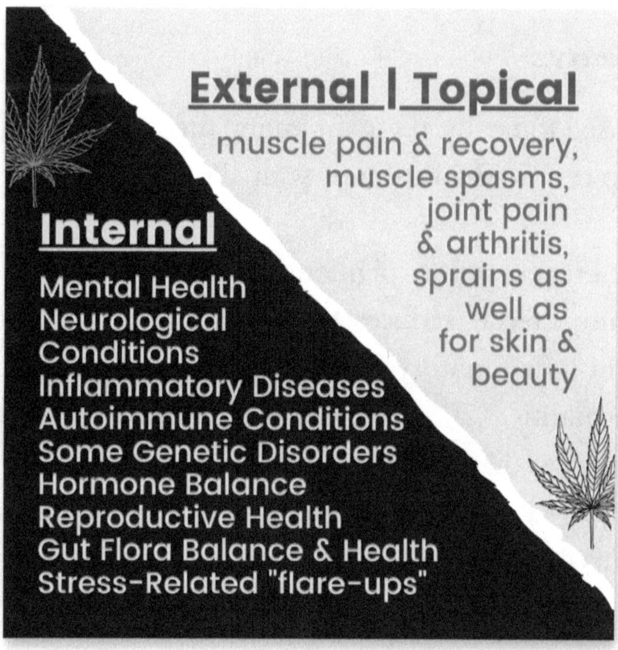


## External Use (Skin, Hair, Muscles, and Joints)

### *Types available*

Salves, balms, creams, hair oils, beard oils, beard balms, skin serums, lotions, body butters, massage or pain-relief gels, roll-ons, bath bombs, bath oils, soaps, lash serums, sunblocks, and massage oils.

***Transdermal patches are also found in this category, but are technically a "hybrid"— a topical application that allows CBD to enter the bloodstream. They carry some internal use risks (such as a positive drug test), but is non-intoxicating, even with higher amounts of THC than hemp offers, and don't carry the risk of medication interaction. They are used for all intents and purposes and function more like an "internal use" product. ***

### *For Beauty*

When used topically, there are many properties of CBD that can help restore the health of your skin, including:

- Cell regeneration (pigmentation, scarring)
- Antibacterial (reduces acne, infections)
- Anti-inflammatory (rosacea, eczema, psoriasis, dermatitis)
- Balances oil production (blackheads, acne)
- Improves collagen production (reduces common signs of aging).

### *Other common uses*

Additional uses for topical CBD include hair growth, muscle and joint pain, bug bites, minor scratches and abrasions, as well as burns, including sunburn.

### *When would it be best to use both?*

Instances where you would want to use it both externally and internally include arthritic joint pain, autoimmune conditions such as psoriasis and rosacea, and acne, since oil production works from the inside out and can often be tied to hormone balance. CBD is not only AWESOME at combating the inflammation that causes muscle and joint pain, but it can also affect our skin condition. Do you struggle with IBS, gastritis, or colitis? These are also inflammatory conditions. When your digestive system is inflamed, nutrients can't be properly absorbed into your bloodstream. Nutrient deficiencies can manifest as skin abnormalities—rashes, discoloration, and/or flaking. A large majority of those who use CBD topically would benefit even more from internal use or from the combination of using both.

### *How much to use?*

External use is pretty straightforward. However, sometimes people unintentionally overuse it. Only use a small amount where it is needed.

A concentration of 100+ mg CBD per oz is a good rule of thumb for high-quality products. Typically, 10-25 mg of CBD (per use/application) is an effective amount for topical relief, as needed. More is not better, nor is it worse. However, using more than is necessary would be a waste of product and money.

***For hair (or beard) growth.***

Using 3 mg of CBD per day, massaged into the scalp or face for 6 months, showed SIGNIFICANT results for both men and women in a large research study on alopecia.

***What to Be Aware Of***

- High-quality topicals will often not include ANY mineral oils, parabens, petroleum products, artificial colors, and fragrances (listed as "fragrance") or any SLS.
- There are healthy ingredients that become counterproductive when used with CBD because they hold properties that "protect" the skin, thus blocking the absorption of the CBD. These include beeswax, coconut oil (in solid form), cocoa butter (if it is the predominant ingredient), marula oil, and moringa oil. As a general rule, if it clogs your pores, the CBD can't reach the receptors.
- CBD products that are "washed" off the skin, such as soaps, shampoos, and body washes, are a bit of a waste, in my opinion. You want the CBD to stay and absorb into the skin receptors. If you are using a salt or sugar scrub, be sure to lightly rinse the exfoliant off, but try to massage in any residual oils to fully utilize the CBD in the product.

***Pros/Cons***

Pros: No risk of medication interaction, no side effects,

easy and discreet to use, a variety of products and price points, no drug testing risks, can be used during pregnancy and breastfeeding, and can be used on children and babies (see the "Pet" section for potential pet usage).

Cons: When using a topical product for pain relief, the effects often only last for an hour or two. If you tolerate essential oils well, look for products using high-quality essential oils (EOs) that boast therapeutic benefits in the ingredients list. The effects of the CBD will be enhanced by the EOs and last longer. Know that "Lavender fragrance" ≠ "Lavender essential oil."

## Internal use

For internal use, we need to break this down even further.

If you are a "healthy" individual and not on any medications, and you want to maintain a strong immune system, healthy digestion, reduce oxidative stress and damage, and prevent age-related diseases and disorders, ANY form of hemp-derived CBD product can benefit you when used internally.

- Read the descriptions of the types (full spectrum, broad spectrum, or isolate) to determine which will fit your lifestyle best.
- Don't forget, if you get drug tested, have any mental health considerations, are pregnant (we will

go more into this), or are using it for your pet, opt for a CBD isolate product.

### *Types available*

Methods of internal use include tinctures (alcohol-based), CBD oils (oil-based sublingual drops), vapes (both dry herb and concentrates), smoking, edibles, chewing gum, transdermal patches, nasal sprays, eye drops, suppositories (both anal and vaginal), toothpaste, mouthwash, pills, drinks, and the list goes on!

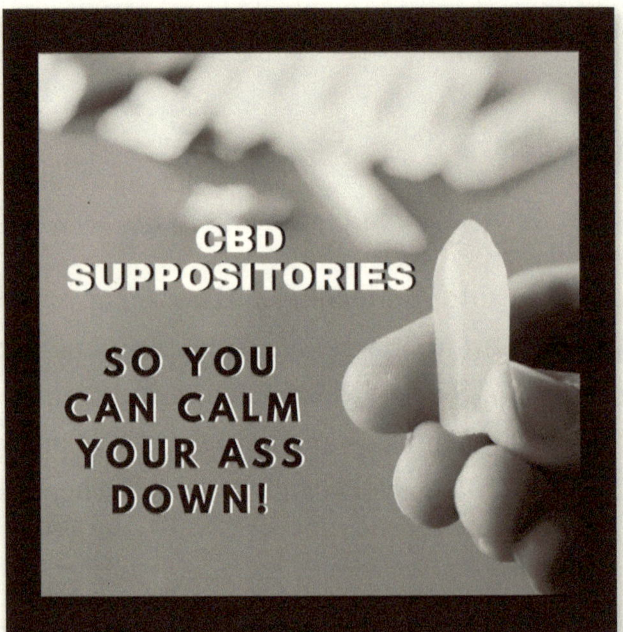


### *Finding your ideal dose, a.k.a. the "sweet spot"*

Hemp-derived CBD is a safe and forgiving supplement. Since there is not yet a standard dosage and each person's biochemistry is unique, it usually takes some trial and error to find your perfect dosage. A good place to start is 1-6 mg per 10 lbs of body weight, based on symptom levels, metabolism, and condition or goals. Maintain the dosage for 5-7 days before adjusting amounts, either up or down. It is best used daily (for preventative purposes) or more than twice a day for health challenges, within 30 minutes of eating. Keep in mind that different methods of ingestion have different onsets, durations, and *bioavailability*.

***Bioavailability*** *is how much of a product—in this case, CBD—that actually enters the bloodstream to be utilized by the body.*

Most CBD products on the market come in low to medium "strengths." I commonly see 5-50 mg of CBD per serving in products at health food stores, in supplement sections, at wellness spas, and/or chiropractor's offices (reputable places where you can purchase CBD). A 5 mg edible is an EXTREMELY low amount for a full-grown adult, especially when you take into account how much of it actually gets utilized by the body after second-pass digestion.

I see a LOT of people get discouraged by this without even knowing that this is the reason the product "didn't work" for them. The most popular "discreet" and easy methods to take CBD are through oral ingestion—gummies, capsules, drinks, or in another form of edible.

The downfall of this method, however, is that it has the LOWEST bioavailability of ALL the ways to take cannabinoids, since it has to pass through the stomach and liver prior to reaching your bloodstream. A majority (6-9%) of the CBD is "lost" in the process and never actually reaches the bloodstream!

Ex: 25 mg CBD gummy = 1.5 mg - 2.25 mg CBD is actually being absorbed!

There are many safe and effective ways to supplement with CBD, but I find natural CBD Oils to be the best fit for me, personally. This way, you are in complete control of the dose, unlike pre-dosed capsules or pre-portioned foods and candies. There are usually no "fillers" that aggravate my condition (e.g., gluten, sugar, artificial colors, and flavors), and the bioavailability of *sublingual* ingestion is significantly higher than that of oral ingestion.

***Sublingual*** *ingestion is when an oil, tincture, or spray is held under the tongue (usually for one minute or more) before swallowing, in order to absorb through the mucous membranes. This bypasses the liver initially, so more (35-45%) CBD reaches the bloodstream.*

| Bioavailability | Onset | Duration |
|---|---|---|
| Sublingual (oils, tinctures, & sprays) 35-45% | 10-20 min. | 4-6 hrs. |
| Oral (Pills, Candies, Edibles, Drinks) 6-9% | 30-120 min. | 4-8 hrs. |
| Aerosol/Nasal 35% | 10-20 min. | 4-6 hrs.. |
| Vape or smoking 30-60% | 0-5 min. | 2-3 hrs. |
| Gums, lozenges 15-30% | 20-40 min. | 4-6 hrs. |
| Suppositories 25-50% | 5-15 min. | 4-8 hrs.. |

## *What to Be Aware Of*

### Medication interactions – *all internal use CBD products*

CBD can alter the way your body processes certain medications, such as pharmaceuticals that interact with the cytochrome P450 pathway.

There are many medications that are processed through the same receptors that CBD utilizes. This means there is a good chance that when the medication or the CBD is taken, it becomes a "first come, first served" situation. Whichever substance reaches the receptors first "wins" and can "work." The other one either gets flushed out of the body and rendered ineffective, or could even increase the risk of side effects of that drug by increasing the levels of said medication in the bloodstream; with the receptors blocked, it will just recirculate through the blood.

There are also some medications that CBD may interact with, which it may enhance. Blood thinners, anti-epileptics, immunosuppressants, and benzodiazepines are some examples of medications that, if you are already taking them and want to incorporate CBD, either to enhance or eventually replace, you should consult with a knowledgeable doctor first. Dosages may need to be adjusted and monitored carefully.

Please work with your doctor, integrative health practitioner, or naturopath before starting or stopping any medications or using CBD at the same time as any prescriptions that caution you to avoid grapefruit juice, St. John's Wort, watercress, or goldenseal. This also applies if you are unsure whether your medication is metabolized by the CYP450 system. *See Appendix I for a list of the most common medication interactions.*

## Side effects

Besides medication interactions, possible side effects (most commonly from high doses of 10-50 mg/kg orally) of CBD could potentially include dry mouth, fatigue, diarrhea, appetite loss, lower blood pressure, and drowsiness. Alcohol use may increase these risks.

To mitigate these side effects, break up your dosage throughout the day (known as "microdosing") in order to obtain optimal energy levels at higher doses. Another option —just take a lower dose. Always listen to your body.

- *High-dose example for oral consumption: 675–3,405 mg CBD per day.*

*This is the equivalent of eating 2 to 6 months' worth of CBD gummies in one sitting!*

- *Keep in mind that these are side effects experienced in clinical research settings, so the CBD may have been in synthetic form.*

Contrary to popular belief—ahem, a misleading article done by a popular online news outlet several years back—CBD does NOT cause liver failure or injury. In fact, studies show that CBD supports liver health and function by reducing inflammation, lowering oxidative stress and fibrosis, and promoting overall liver function. Animal studies suggest that CBD can also alleviate liver damage caused by alcohol consumption and a high-fat diet.

## Addiction, overdose, and tolerance.

CBD is non-addictive; there have been no known overdoses or deaths related to CBD. Although individual experiences may vary, CBD is known to have a *reverse tolerance or sensitiza-*

*tion* effect. This means that it takes *less CBD over time to achieve the same benefits* as one once had when using higher doses.

Since our bodies make cannabinoids, we are essentially "refilling" our bodies with the cannabinoids needed to function optimally. Once our bodies start hitting that high-functioning level, the only time we would need cannabinoid levels "refilled" is when we are enduring a period of high stress, trauma, injury, or an ongoing degenerative issue. Typically, once a condition becomes cured or stable, one can often stop taking CBD or remain on a lower, preventative "maintenance" dose.

*When I started taking CBD for my health issues, I found my "sweet spot" at 80-90 mg/day. (For reference, I was a 125 lb woman with a moderate metabolism.) As symptoms started improving, I began reducing the amount I took to 50-60 mg/day. After about 18 months, I felt good enough to reduce that amount to 25-35 mg/day (unless I was in a "flare," in which case I would bump it up temporarily). I still take CBD to this day, but I am doing so preventively. I now take 25 mg/day (in CBD oil form—sublingually), but usually only 3–4 days a week in the summer; I take more in the winter when my pain levels get higher.*

## CBD for Special Populations: FAQs"

### Can I use CBD during pregnancy?

CBD is commonly used for pregnancy-related symptoms, including nausea, insomnia, anxiety, and chronic pain. Although there is no comprehensive research (human studies) on its safety during pregnancy, a few rat and mouse studies were conducted to test the impact of CBD, THC, and 1:1 THC:CBD in prenatal rodents. The effects on the offspring are as follows:

- The findings varied and were often sex-specific. Female rodents were at higher risk of having offspring with more anxiety and a higher capacity for complex problem solving. *Ignorance is bliss," right?!* Males, with low-dose gestational exposure to CBD, showed increased body weight.
- We DO know that both cannabinoids, THC and CBD, pass through the placenta as well as through breast milk.
- Frequent Cannabis use during pregnancy is attributed to low birth weights, with THC, and was inconclusive for CBD without THC.
- Most pregnant women seek advice on cannabis use during pregnancy—from dispensary employees to family and friends. Because of this, more studies and education are needed! More often than not, the women are seeking a "safer" alternative to prescription medications. When weighing the risks, CBD often comes out on top.
- The studies varied among human studies; there were a variety of amounts and forms of maternal cannabis use (from light to heavy usage), including cannabis cigarettes. Along with this, some mothers were co-using with other substances. The

> participants came from varying cultures, ethnicities, and socioeconomic standings.

All in all, there isn't enough research available on the topic regarding CBD only during pregnancy. However, THC use is discouraged due to potential neurodevelopmental risks, as stated in Chapter 15.

## Ranger's Tale

It was the last day of elementary school in June for our two children. We had casually talked about getting another dog about six months after our beloved Golden Retriever, Jake, had passed away. Here we were, a few years later, settled into a new home with a fenced yard in a very pet-friendly neighborhood.

We knew we didn't have the time or patience to train a puppy. We had really enjoyed getting Jake as a rescue. He was already housebroken and was past that chewing-on-everything-they-can-get-ahold-of stage, so that experience opened our eyes to adoption. Knowing that the local no-kill shelters were overflowing with incoming pets from other states made it an easy decision for us to at least "look" at a potential new member of our family.

We weren't in a hurry. We just wanted the right fit for our lifestyle. Ideally, a lazy, housebroken, large dog that would be both protective of our little family and great with kids. As a family, we met several dogs that were available at our local humane society. They were all nice, but some were high energy, and some had no interest whatsoever in interacting with our kiddos. Others would whine incessantly (poor things), and a few were hiding—just terrified.

As we headed to the exit, we saw Wesley. He eagerly saw us approaching and pressed his black nose through the bars to be seen. His entire 65 lb, tall but lean pit bull mix frame wiggled violently in unison with the wag of his whip-like tail. My kids immediately picked up on his signal—that he was just longing to be touched. They quickly reached their arms through the bars to give him a good ear scratch before we could say, "The sign says to keep away from the gates."

It was too late. They were already in love with the white pittie mix, with large brindle spots, including a patch over one eye. He was pressing his entire body against the bars to receive the maximum amount of petting possible. I glanced up at his paperwork. He had been shipped to Spokane, WA, from Houston, Texas, the day before. He was approximately 3 years old, housebroken, good with kids and other dogs (cats were questionable), but most importantly, a BIG black placard above it all read "RESERVED - ADOPTED."

"Sorry, kids, not this one. He isn't even available."

"Can we just have them get a leash so we can play with him in the dog yard?" asked my eight-year-old son.

They didn't allow it. It was drawing close to closing time, so, grasping at straws, I asked the staff member if she could call me if his adoption fell through.

"They have 24 hours to get him once the reserved sign goes up, and they just left an hour ago," she said. Quoting Lloyd from *Dumb and Dumber*, I jokingly exclaimed, "So you're telling me there's a chance!"

Lucky for us, we got a call the next day. Wesley was in rough shape. His paws were cracked and bleeding in some spots. His skin and fur were patchy, red, and irritated. He cried the whole way home in his new crate, filled with soft blankets and new chew toys. As soon as we got to the house, he bounced between each member of the family to get affection. All the while, the end of his tail was whacking walls and furniture while spurting blood profusely. We soon found out it was called "Happy Tail Syndrome." Unfortunately, it wasn't as fun as it sounds and made our living room look like a scene out of *Dexter*. He didn't seem to notice, though.

He discovered our backyard and made himself at home, marking his territory and doing "zoomies" around the apple tree while intermittently "checking on" the kids. As a way to welcome him to the family, we agreed on renaming him Ranger since he was from Texas (we expected Chuck Norris-like "badassery" from him).

Our local vet helped us nurse Ranger back to health; we discovered his allergies (food and environmental) and were able to make the changes needed. The vet also estimated his age to be between 12 and 18 months old due to his still having some baby teeth.

"You mean he's still growing?" we asked.

Yep.

By the time he was pushing 100 lbs, about 3 to 4 months later, Ranger had settled nicely into our family's routine. He had started filling out, gaining quite a bit of muscle, and had become quite spoiled. He had his own dedicated spot on the couch, a toy box filled with fun activities to keep him busy, and a couple of outfits that kept him warm in our colder climate. He had found his groove—casually rolling out of my son's bed around 7 a.m., greeting us for breakfast (eating his homemade dog food), and doing a few zoomies around the coffee table or around the apple trees if the weather was nice. He'd then settle in on the couch for an afternoon nap after some ear scratches and additional snuggles until Dad came home from work and took him on his afternoon run. He led a pretty charmed life.

It was right around this time when he started having seizures. At first, we didn't even know what was going on. He would just sit oddly still, and his head would shake—usually with his eyes closed. Afterwards, he would act confused or whimper.

We told our vet what was going on. It was a couple of months after he had his first seizure (that we knew of) before a second one occurred. Then a third one, only three weeks later. We realized that not only were they happening more frequently, but they were also lasting longer. It was scary.

At that point in my career, I had already been studying cannabis medicine independently for almost 4 years and had created my own brand of Hemp CBD products that I formulated, manufactured, and retailed as a side hustle for two years.

I was well aware of the benefits of CBD for people with epilepsy (seizure disorders). I also knew that since dogs are built differently than we are, I had to make sure that if I was going to attempt to make a product for him, I would have to do my research to ensure it was safe and effective.

After quickly learning all that I could on the subject, which I will share in the next section, I developed a CBD pet oil. I kept it close to Ranger's favorite spot on the couch, just in case he had another seizure.

Of course he wasn't in "his spot" when the seizure came the first time, after being ready for it, so I rushed over to grab the CBD and squeezed a dropperful into his cheek. The seizing stopped immediately. I chalked it up to getting there too late. I wasn't sure if it worked or if it was just going to stop anyway.

About a month passed before it happened again. Ranger was "in his spot," and the CBD bottle and I were only an arm's reach away. About five seconds into the seizure, I was able to administer the oil, and it instantly stopped. At this point, the seizures had been lasting anywhere from one to three minutes. I realized it wasn't a coincidence; the CBD really worked to stop his seizures. What a blessing!

Now that I knew it was effective at treating seizures, I wanted to see if it could prevent them as well. After learning that it was safe to give pets CBD daily, I started adding it to his dog food—morning and night. No more seizures.

It was just over a year before Ranger had another seizure. We had gone on vacation, and when packing Ranger's bag for his pet sitter's place, we failed to stock him with enough CBD oil for the length of our trip. Two days before our return, the pet sitter ran out of the drops for Ranger.

When we returned home and brought him back to the house, he started having a seizure. I scrambled through Ranger's bag—not knowing yet that he had run out while we were gone. Unfortunate as that was, it led us to realize two things:

1. The CBD oil was actively preventing the seizures.

2. It lasted in his system for a couple of days before it was no longer preventing them.

As I am typing this, it has been over six years since Ranger's last seizure. He is "helping me" type this in the picture below. He became the "poster boy" for Herb 'N Oil's pet line. Although I have since shut down the retail business, I still make CBD for Ranger at home.

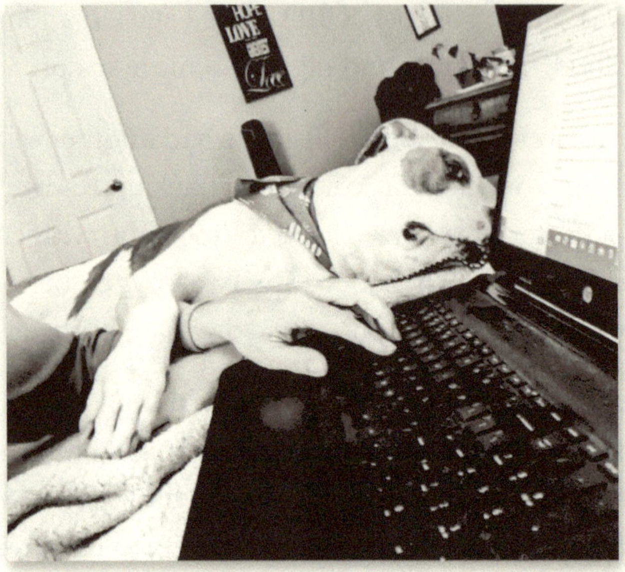

## CBD for Pets

Almost all animals have an endocannabinoid system, including birds, mammals, reptiles, fish, and even some invertebrates (such as sea urchins, worms, and mussels). Now, I am not a holistic veterinarian, but I do understand some basics about the endocannabinoid systems of many household pets and livestock animals, including dogs, cats, parakeets, horses, goats, cows, rabbits, and sheep. I grew up on a ranch, remember?

Over time, I had the honor of sharing my knowledge and products with various businesses in the "pet and vet" community. Since studies, and therefore education, on CBD for pets are limited, a majority of the information comes from the properties of CBD and how it interacts with the animal's body through case studies, anecdotal evidence, and what I call "educated connections."

*For example:*

*Knowing that CBD has very strong anti-inflammatory properties and helps reduce joint inflammation, relieve pain, and improve mobility in dogs with arthritis, it would be safe, and presumably correct (according to all the veterinarians I have consulted with), to assume that it will also help with tendon inflammation, relieve pain, and improve mobility in dogs with tendonitis.*

There are several common questions that I am frequently asked about cannabis and/or hemp use in animals. The following are the most common things that people want to know.

**What is CBD used for, and can it help my pet?**

CBD can help your pet with wound healing, systemic inflammation (such as arthritis), seizures, cancer, post-surgical recovery, improved sleep, pain relief, and anxiety. Many of the same things CBD can help us with, it can also help your pet with.

Anxious behaviors in pets can look like, but aren't limited to, pacing, panting, drooling, excessive digging or other destructive behavior, changes in sleeping patterns, changes in appetite, and excessive noise-making. Keep in mind that CBD is NOT a substitute for exercise, seeking medical attention, proper training, or love and affection.

### Why can't my pet have just any CBD or medical cannabis product?

It is best for pets to avoid products with any THC in them. This includes the small amount of THC that is naturally occurring in hemp CBD products. Animals have a very limited number of CB1 receptors, so they become overloaded (extremely intoxicated) with just the smallest amount of THC. THC free products are the only safe way to use cannabis for animals. In fact, many local veterinarians struggle with pets overdosing on recreational and medical cannabis products that the owner has left within reach of the pet or has negligently fed their pet—either for "fun" or with good intentions to help a condition.

### Is CBD legal for pets? If so, why is pet CBD hard to find?

Even though Hemp CBD is federally legal, it is state-regulated. This includes the rules and laws for animal use. Some states differentiate "pets" from "livestock" and "veterinary" use. The National Animal Supplement Council (NASC) verifies the safety and efficacy of CBD in dogs and notes that it is well tolerated. Of course, the American Veterinary Medical Association (AVMA) claims that there "isn't enough scientific evidence to suggest that it can help dogs." CBD products (along with fish oil, glucosamine, and other common supplements) are not FDA-approved.

### How do I choose a product that is right for my pet?

Like "for people" products, you want to look for third-party testing from reputable brands and knowledgeable sellers. Make sure the product is THC free (0% THC, not full spectrum). Just because a product is *made* for pets doesn't mean the product is *safe* for pets. I have seen countless bottles and packages of products with THC in them at pet stores—well-intentioned but misinformed.

**How much do I give my pet?**

This varies greatly by type of animal, type of issue, and severity of condition. Ranger takes 25 mg CBD isolate tincture twice daily, morning and night, with food, and he is a 100 lb dog with epilepsy. One customer with a very anxious cockatiel gave her bird a 15 mg CBD isolate salmon treat once daily, with great success. The most common suggested use is 1-3 mg per kg. (Example: A 20 lb pet would take anywhere from 9-30 mg CBD.) CBD typically lasts in the system for about 6 to 8 hours, since it is usually easiest just to feed the pet CBD. With people and rats, it is up to 4 times more effective when taken within 30 minutes of eating. It's safe to assume the same for pets.

**What about risks, side effects, and medication interactions?**

The highest risk comes from the potential THC in a pet product. THC can not only get your pet high, but it can also be toxic for them, making them very sick. It is rarely lethal, although it could cause vomiting, drooling, seizures, disorientation, lethargy, incontinence, and even put them in a coma. If your pet has ingested THC, seek immediate veterinary care.

Medication interactions with pets are the same as in people. www.Whole-Dog-Journal.com does a good job of explaining the nuances of potential medication interactions for dogs, but the principles apply to all animals with an ECS. If the medication relies on P450 enzymes to metabolize, CBD could interact with it in one way or another. It enhances the effects of some medications and blocks the effects of others, so ask your vet or a knowledgeable CBD consultant before using it with other medicines.

If there is no THC in the product and there are no other medications being taken with it, the side effects are minimal, if any. It may make the animal drowsy and may also have detoxifying qualities (minor or short-term stool softening or potential diarrhea) in higher doses. Even at higher doses, it is not lethal, addictive, or dangerous.

## How did we get here?

Throughout time, cannabis has been used as medicine, in ceremony, and steeped in tradition. As U.S. government leaders saw the potential for it to replace the new commodities in which they were vested, they demonized it in order to control its future. By discrediting herbal medicine and building out the processes of standardization, medical education, and reliance on petroleum products, leaders of the time were not only able to gain significant profits through this course of action, but it also allowed them to control what was being taught to future generations. They stirred up fear through lies with racist ties. They preyed on the poor, the immigrants, the women, and the underserved populations. They teamed up and helped fund a media empire to spread fear and lies in order to control the narrative.

Cannabis, hemp, marijuana—a plant with so many uses, untapped potential, and endless healing properties—got in the way of wealth and control. I don't think it is a miracle plant, though many do. I don't think it's the end-all, be-all, though many do. I think we should have the right to choose to use it if we wish. I think we should have access to the truth about the plant and the history of why it was demonized. I think that education about the plant should be widespread, devoid of biases from both sides.

I think the industry deserves to be heard—in a real way. Cannabis businesses are still highly restricted in their ability to reach their true potential. They are restricted by the FDA, the medical community, and the federal and state governments. They are being filtered, banned, and censored by social media, web hosting platforms, and major commerce and commercial media sites. The restricted access to banking and transportation is killing off well-intentioned businesses right and left. The taxes, insurance, and permitting in most regulated areas are keeping growers, dispensaries, and manufacturers in a tight spot financially.

Meanwhile, people are waking up. They are seeing all the

ways we have been lied to. They are realizing that pharmacology is not necessarily the path to health. There is a form of cannabis for everyone: struggling moms, military veterans, men working hard daily through chronic pain, children with epilepsy, entrepreneurs with ADHD, grandparents with arthritis, college students with autoimmune diseases, doctors struggling with sobriety, celebrities with performance anxiety, athletes in surgical rehab, and teens with depression, to name a few.

By understanding how our bodies work with the cannabinoids found in cannabis in order to regain wellness, we can now take control of our own health. We can make smart decisions by supporting our endocannabinoid systems through a mindful lifestyle—supporting our emotional and spiritual health and limiting the toxins with which we are inundated on a daily basis.

The fear that was once ingrained in us is now giving way to the hope that cannabis could bring to those most in need. The truth is coming out. We are telling the tale of taking the path less traveled—the path of healing the way God intended: through faith, forgiveness, food, and herbs.

# WORKS CITED


- "A History of the FDA and Drug Regulation in the United States." *U.S. Food and Drug Administration*, www.fda.gov/sentennial/history/history.html. Accessed 20 July 2025.
- Al-Ghezi, Zaidon Z., et al. "Combination of Cannabinoids, Delta-9-Tetrahydrocannabinol (THC) and Cannabidiol (CBD), Mitigates Experimental Autoimmune Encephalomyelitis (EAE) by Altering the Gut Microbiome." Brain, Behavior, and Immunity, vol. 82, 2019, pp. 25–35. https://doi.org/10.1016/j.bbi.2019.07.028.
- Barbosa-Leiker, Celestina, et al. "Daily Cannabis Use During Pregnancy and Postpartum in a State with Legalized Recreational Cannabis." Journal of Addiction Medicine, vol. 14, no. 6, 2020, pp. 467–474. https://doi.org/10.1097/ADM.0000000000000625.
- Cooper, Ziva D., and Rebecca M. Craft. "Sex-Dependent Effects of Cannabis and Cannabinoids: A Translational Perspective." Neuroscience & Biobehavioral Reviews, vol. 97, 2018, pp. 19–34. https://doi.org/10.1016/j.neubiorev.2018.01.003.
- Craft, R. M., et al. "Sex Differences in Cannabinoid Pharmacology: A Reflection of Differences in the Endocannabinoid System?" Neuropharmacology, vol. 65, 2013, pp. 49–57. https://doi.org/10.1016/j.neuropharm.2012.07.019.
- Ellermann, Miriam. "Emerging Mechanisms by Which Endocannabinoids and Their Derivatives Modulate Bacterial Populations within the Gut Microbiome." Advances in Drug and

Alcohol Research, vol. 3, 2023, Article 11359. https://doi.org/10.3389/adar.2023.11359.

- ElSohly, Mahmoud A., et al. "Changes in Cannabis Potency over the Last 2 Decades (1995–2014): Analysis of Current Data in the United States." Biological Psychiatry, vol. 79, no. 7, 2016, pp. 613–619. https://doi.org/10.1016/j.biopsych.2016.01.004.
- Fakhoury, Marc. "Role of the Endocannabinoid System in the Pathophysiology of Schizophrenia." *Molecular Neurobiology*, vol. 54, no. 1, 2017, pp. 768–778. https://doi.org/10.1007/s12035-016-9697-5.
- Fattore, Liana, and Walter Fratta. "How Important Are Sex Differences in Cannabinoid Action?" Progress in Neuro-Psychopharmacology and Biological Psychiatry, vol. 34, no. 4, 2010, pp. 633–648. https://doi.org/10.1016/j.pnpbp.2010.07.006.
- Freeman, Tom P., et al. "Cannabidiol for the Treatment of Cannabis Use Disorder: A Phase 2a, Double-Blind, Placebo-Controlled, Randomised, Adaptive Bayesian Trial." The Lancet Psychiatry, vol. 7, no. 10, 2020, pp. 865–874. https://doi.org/10.1016/S2215-0366(20)30290-X.
- Gamble, L. J., et al. "Pharmacokinetics, Safety, and Clinical Efficacy of Cannabidiol Treatment in Osteoarthritic Dogs." *Frontiers in Veterinary Science*, vol. 5, 2018, p. 165.
- Hill, Matthew N., et al. "The Role of the Endocannabinoid System in the Regulation of the Hypothalamic-Pituitary-Adrenal Axis and Emotional Stress." Psychoneuroendocrinology, vol. 32, no. 8–10, 2007, pp. 1043–1059. https://doi.org/10.1016/j.psychres.2007.01.006.
- Iezzi, Daniela, et al. "In Utero Exposure to Cannabidiol Disrupts Select Early-Life Behaviors in a Sex-Specific Manner." Translational Psychiatry, vol. 12, no. 1, 2022, article 501. https://doi.org/10.1038/s41398-022-02271-8.
- Khalid, Nadeem, et al. "Cannabis Versus Opioids for Pain."

StatPearls, StatPearls Publishing, 2024. https://www.ncbi.nlm.nih.gov/books/NBK573080/.

- Kathuria, S., et al. "Modulation of Anxiety through Blockade of Anandamide Hydrolysis." Nature Medicine, vol. 9, 2003, pp. 76–81. https://doi.org/10.1038/nm803.
- Kogan, L. R., Hellyer, P. W., and Robinson, N. G. "Consumers' Perceptions of Hemp Products for Animals." Journal of the American Holistic Veterinary Medical Association, no. 52, 2019, pp. 16–26.
- Lee, Soo Yeun, et al. "Estrogenic Effects of Marijuana Smoke Condensate and Cannabinoid Compounds." Toxicology and Applied Pharmacology, vol. 208, no. 1, 2005, pp. 43–50. https://www.sciencedirect.com/science/article/abs/pii/S0041008X06000093.
- "Chemist Creates Aspirin and Heroin." Pharmacy Times, https://www.pharmacytimes.com/view/chemist-creates-aspirin-and-heroin. Accessed 20 July 2025.
- "History of Marijuana Regulation in the United States - Marijuana Law in the United States." University of Georgia School of Law, https://search.app/JfahbEnqnZKXMTCr8. Accessed 20 July 2025.
- "Mel Frank – Cannabis Plant Anatomy." BeyondTHC.com, https://beyondthc.com. Accessed 20 July 2025.
- "Molecular Targets of Cannabinoids: A Focused Review on CBD." BioSource Botanicals, https://biosourcebotanicals.com/molecular-targets-of-cannabinoids-a-focused-review-on-cbd/. Accessed 20 July 2025.
- Rubio-Tapia, Alberto, et al. "AGA Clinical Practice Update on Diagnosis and Management of Cannabinoid Hyperemesis Syndrome: Commentary." 1 May 2024.
- "Salicylic Acid from Salicin: The Birth of Modern Pain Relief." PubMed Central, https://www.ncbi.nlm.nih.gov/pmc/articles/PMC1894700/. Accessed 20 July 2025.

- "Timeline 1925–1945." Bayer, https://www.bayer.com/en/history/1925-1945. Accessed 20 July 2025.
- "CBD Statistics." Mastermind Behavior, https://www.mastermindbehavior.com/post/cbd-statistics. Accessed 20 July 2025.
- Books Cited
- Chopra, Deepak, and Rudolph E. Tanzi. *Super Genes: Unlock the Astonishing Power of Your DNA for Optimum Health and Well-Being*. Harmony Books, 2015.
- Conrad, Chris. *Hemp for Health: The Medicinal and Nutritional Uses of Cannabis Sativa*. Healing Arts Press, 1997.
- Sansouci, Jenny. *The Rebel's Apothecary: A Practical Guide to the Healing Magic of Cannabis, CBD, and Mushrooms*. Harper Wave, 2020.
- Danielle Simone Brand. *Weed Mom: The Canna-Curious Woman's Guide to Healthier Relaxation, Happier Parenting, and Chilling TF Out*. Ulysses Press, 2021.
- Leinow, Leonard, and Juliana Birnbaum. *CBD: A Patient's Guide to Medicinal Cannabis—Healing Without the High*. North Atlantic Books, 2017.
- Lee, Martin A. *Smoke Signals: A Social History of Marijuana - Medical, Recreational and Scientific*. Scribner, 2012.

## OTHER RECOMMENDED READING


- Black, Paula and Captain Dale *Life, Cancer and God: Healing Your Body, Soul, and Spirit*. Black Eagle Publishing, 2014.
- Burg, Bob, and John David Mann. *The Go-Giver: A Little Story About a Powerful Business Idea*. Portfolio, 2007.
- Clear, James. *Atomic Habits*. Avery, 2018.
- Colbert, Don. *The 7 Pillars of Health: The Natural Way to Better Health for Life*. Siloam Press, 2007.


1. spanish slang for a small, personal amount of cannabis ↑
2. For hemp recipes, CBD meals, and to enhance your daily diet by using culinary terpenes, be sure to sign up for my recipe newsletter, "Cooking with Buds." ↑

# APPENDIX I

Medications that can be affected by CBD (including isolate)

CBD inhibits CYP3A4, CYP2D6, and CYP2C9.

This can increase blood levels of many drugs or reduce the activation of pro-drugs.

> CBD = inhibitor of:

CYP3A4 (strong)

CYP2D6 (moderate–strong)

CYP2C19 (moderate)

CYP2C9 (moderate)

1. Medications Affected by CYP3A4 Inhibition

(CBD slows their breakdown → higher drug levels)

- Antidepressants: Sertraline (Zoloft), Citalopram / Escitalopram, Venlafaxine, Trazodone
- Antihistamines: Loratadine (Claritin), Cetirizine (minor)

- Benzodiazepines: Alprazolam, Clonazepam, Midazolam, Triazolam
- Opioids: Oxycodone, Fentanyl, Methadone, Buprenorphine
- Cardiac & Blood Pressure: Amlodipine, Diltiazem, Verapamil, Atorvastatin, Simvastatin, Lovastatin
- Immunosuppressants: Tacrolimus, Cyclosporine, Sirolimus
- Steroids: Prednisone / Prednisolone (minor), Dexamethasone (minor)
- Others: Sildenafil (Viagra), Buspirone, Ketamine

2. Medications Affected via CYP2D6 Inhibition

(CBD slows breakdown → increased drug levels)

- Antidepressants: Fluoxetine(Prozac), Paroxetine, Duloxetine, Bupropion, Amitriptyline and other TCAs
- Antipsychotics: Risperidone, Haloperidol, Aripiprazole, Olanzapine (also 1A2)
- Opioids - whose activation depends on CYP2D6 (CBD may reduce effectiveness of these): Codeine → less conversion into morphine, Tramadol → less active metabolite, Hydrocodone (partial), Oxycodone (partial)
- Cardiac medications: Metoprolol, Propranolol

3. Medications Affected via CYP2C19 Inhibition

(CBD slows breakdown OR activation)

- SSRIs: Citalopram, Escitalopram, Sertraline (secondary)
- Benzodiazepines: Diazepam
- Blood thinner: Clopidogrel — CBD may reduce activation, causing reduced effect
- GI meds: Omeprazole (Prilosec), Esomeprazole, Lansoprazole

4. Medications Affected via CYP2C9 Inhibition

- Blood thinner: Warfarin — CBD can significantly raise INR
- NSAIDs: Ibuprofen, Naproxen (Aleve), Diclofenac (Voltaren)
- Diabetes meds: Glipizide, Glyburide
- Seizure meds: Phenytoin

5. Medications Affected via UGT Inhibition (less known but important)

CBD also inhibits UGT1A9 and UGT2B7, affecting: Morphine, Lorazepam, Oxcarbazepine, Zidovudine (HIV), Valproic acid

www.ingramcontent.com/pod-product-compliance
Lightning Source LLC
LaVergne TN
LVHW100259210926
848480LV00003B/963

* 9 7 9 8 9 0 2 2 2 8 9 8 1 *